Infinity
in a Box

Infinity in a Box

Using Yoga to Live with EASE

Megan McDonough

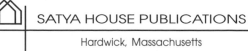
SATYA HOUSE PUBLICATIONS

Hardwick, Massachusetts

Published in the United States of America
by Satya House Publications
P. O. Box 272
Hardwick, Massachusetts 01037
www.satyahouse.com

Manufactured in Canada

First Edition

ISBN 0-9729191-0-4

Cover and book design by Julie Murkette
Cover art by Chuck Kidd

To Mom
for life, love and lemonade

Acknowledgments

When I began this book too many years ago, I naively thought that writing was a solo adventure. I hunched over a keyboard, the writer would tap out ideas that bubbled up from a deep well of creativity. My experience couldn't have been further from the romanticized version.

Rather than a one-person show, the book came to life through everyday relationships, through those generous enough to share their insights, and from the many and varied back and forth dialogs of friends, family and acquaintances.

Ideas came from a wide swath of interactions. Though impossible to acknowledge all, I'm going to give it a shot.

First, to my insanely supportive husband and my ever-flexible children: you are my anchor and the wind in my sails.

To my first Yoga teacher, Nancy Nowak of The Centered Place, whose commitment to Yoga and in-depth expertise gave me an incredibly strong foundation. To Dr. V. S. Rao, founding Director of the High Tech Yoga Institute where I received my Yoga teacher certification. To the countless Yoga teachers who have inspired me with their work; your contribution to the Yoga community and the world at large enhances us all.

To Gen Kelsang Chöma, whose down-to-earth style of teaching Buddhism has influenced me more than she probably realizes.

To Julie Murkette for her precise and patient editing of the manuscript, and her talented ability to transform plain white paper into a finished book. And, most especially, my gratitude to Julie for her willingness to tackle the cover design in the eleventh hour.

To Catherine Carr for her meticulous review of the manuscript, and to Matt Carr, a technical guru who is always willing to answer my frantic calls for help when my computers act quirky.

To Margaret Marcuson and Kathleen Spivak whose insightful suggestions added depth to the story.

A special thanks to Kathleen Lovenbury, whose artistic talent and warm heart never cease to inspire.

I'm honored to have Chuck Kidd's simple and elegant artwork grace the cover. Thank you Chuck, for your open heart and willingness to play with form, transforming this book into a work of art.

To Michelle DeMarco, who helped me clarify the artistic vision for the cover.

Thank you to Joanne Meehl, a wonderful writer who started and led a local writers' group that was the impetus I needed to start this book. And to Margaret and Karl who were part of that group and enriched me with their writing, as well as their feedback. Who would have guessed where our little writing group would take us?

And finally, thanks to my Yoga students. I have learned so much from you all.

Contents

Introduction

In 1854 Henry David Thoreau wrote in *Walden*, "I went to the woods because I wished to live deliberately, to front only the essential facts of life, and see if I could not learn what it had to teach, and not, when I came to die, discover that I had not lived." Thoreau describes how he spent $28.12 on a ten-by-fifteen-square-foot home and created what can only be called a Spartan lifestyle.

There's an ominous note in Thoreau's words. Nobody wants to go to the grave knowing life was wasted. We all want to live life completely, fully. It's part of our human nature. For most of us, however, our lives are not conducive to such an adventure of isolation as Thoreau's. We're busy earning a living, keeping family responsibilities, and saving for retirement.

There's something very romantic about the notion of escape, but I would miss my king-size bed.

So, here's the question for those of us fully immersed in a typical twenty-first century day: Rather than retreating to the woods, can we live deliberately, here and now, in the circumstances we currently find ourselves?

The answer is a conditional yes. Yes because the essentials are, by definition, always present. The most essential is your indivisible essence, the core of who you are. It's impossible to be separated from it. The yes, however, is conditional because we need much more vigilance to stay focused on the essentials when our busy lives pull and push us off course.

While Thoreau took long walks in the wood, we sit in traffic commuting to work. While Thoreau observed nature for hours, we balance the kids' soccer schedules with our business travel. While Thoreau contemplated the meaning of life, we daydream to escape boredom. Thoreau's existence seems exotic, ours mundane.

What a drag to be so . . . normal.

There is hope, however, to know the essentials and to live deliberately even in a typically predictable twenty-first century day. Living deliberately is a matter of focus, not of surroundings; a matter of choice, not of circumstance; a matter of priority, not of personality.

Why bother to live deliberately? Why add that onto an already too long to-do list? To entertain the idea that your life is worthy of such focused awareness raises the value you place on your own existence. Living deliberately, taking time to notice all the little things in everyday life, is a solid proclamation stating, "I believe my life is important. My life is worthy of my attention. My life is a gift I will not waste." In fact, living deliberately does not mean you have to add another item on your list of things to do, like going to the gym. It's much easier than that. Just take that to-do list and decide to do everything on it with deliberate awareness.

In this busy century it's easy to lose yourself. It's easy to forget who you are and end up with a life filled with never-ending activity.

During the whirlwind a quiet sigh escapes, whispering the questions, "Why bother? What's the sense? Who am I?" Living deliberately answers these questions.

You have thoughts; you are not your thoughts. You have feelings; you are not your feelings. You have your bad habits and your good habits; you are neither of them. You have your sins and your virtues; you are much more than either. You even have a body; you are much more than that image in the mirror. Who you are is much grander than you can imagine. Living deliberately enables you to see, and be, this grander reality of self.

What must it be like to face death knowing that life has not been lived? To know that the opportunity to experience your grandest vision of self is lost? The intent of this book is to help you learn through deliberate living that which your life has to teach. Its purpose is to help you connect with the light within, even, or perhaps especially, in this world so far removed from Thoreau's.

The Work of Yoga

My town's country store doubles as a post office. When I moved here in 1989, mail addressed to me would come "General Delivery" which meant I didn't even have a post office box. I simply went up to the counter, greeted the postmistress, Marcia, who smiled, asked about the family and handed me the mail. It reminded me of days long past where milk, gossip, coffee and mail could be picked up at the same spot. It still does even though I now have an official post office box.

One day on the post office wall I saw a poster for a yoga class, vying for attention amidst the community events, lost puppy signs and free kitten offers. It was only a 45-minute drive, less than the typical 1-hour drive needed to find civilization from this cow-country haven.

I started that Yoga class over ten years ago. I'm still practicing today.

Yoga has become a craze of late. Super-model Christie Turlington is on the cover of *Time* with an incredible pose of strength and flexibility. Madonna tells Oprah how she practices "power Yoga" as her only form of exercise. The ancient art of Yoga meets twenty-first century America.

My Yoga practice has never looked so exotic. Nor has my body ever taken the sculpted appearance of the material girl, much to my chagrin. My body, life and work are much more average.

When I first began Yoga, I was a national accounts manager for a fast-moving healthcare company. I traveled the country weekly, negotiating deals, creating and strengthening relationships, and attending meetings. My weekly Yoga class was a great stress reducer.

I now teach Yoga. One of my students came into class and announced that she had had a dream about me the night before. She said, "In my dream, Megan, you told me to do seventy hours of Yoga every week." I responded, "Why would you only do it seventy hours a week?"

Yoga is not limited to the physical movements. The physical flexibility gained from Yoga is nothing compared to the shift in mental flexibility—the ability to see your world and problems in a new and expanded light.

The word Yoga means "union" or "wholeness." Yoga is not simply postures; it's a way of being, a way of looking at yourself in relation to the world. Why then would you limit your practice to only seventy hours per week?

My first inkling that Yoga could be much more than a stress reducer in my life came when I was expecting my first child. Wanting to spend less time traveling, I found a new job that would keep me closer to home. I landed in a Fortune 50 company very different culturally from the organization I left.

I joined a newly formed team assembled during the early Clinton era, when healthcare was *the* main topic of the day. Every healthcare company, including the one I worked for, was scrambling to address the profound shifts of healthcare delivery. It was the pinnacle of managed care companies, whose high stock price reflected the high hopes that they could save the system and control wild spending.

The basic mission of the team I was part of was to transform the way our company did business in such a mutable landscape. Creating something from nothing with a "dream team"—who could ask for anything more?

Three years later, I did ask for more. I begged for something—anything—even if it was less. Thirty-six months after the group's inception—four reorganizations, six managers, innumerable lists of key customers, and at least four separate strategic plans later—I questioned my sanity. Before the game of musical chairs, I viewed myself as an achiever . . . a go-getter. Now I was no longer able to embrace the view that I was a person who could get things done, since nothing was getting done.

Unable to affect the external reality—trying to do that only led to more frustration—I turned inward. The only other choices I saw were the usual: either leave the company or check out emotionally. I explored both; neither was satisfying.

Sometimes being trapped has advantages. I had no place else to go, so I might as well go inward for sanctuary.

At this point my Yoga practice changed from simply doing postures as a physical workout to an introspective outlook that changed the way I related to work.

A joke I heard on the car radio put my troubles at work in perspective. A comedian was talking about Whisk laundry detergent. "Do you remember what Whisk was especially good at removing?" he asked the audience.

"Ring around the collar!" the audience yelled in unison.

"You scrub, you soak, you bleach those nasty ring-around-the-collar stains and they just don't come out," the comedian said. "It seems to me that if you just WASH YOUR NECK the problem would be solved!"

Life is a little like the Whisk commercial. We spend a whole lot of time scrubbing, soaking, and bleaching our external problems. Why won't this stain in my life come out? We lament. Whether work is a pain, the kids' demands are as high as a millionaire's ransom, or we face one of a gazillion other struggles, we try to fix, cope or at least subdue the irritation.

All we're doing is spending excess energy scrubbing the dirt out of the collar of life rather than simply washing our necks.

The best-kept secret of Yoga is how it changes your relationship between the external world and your internal framework. Yoga continually expands your awareness by training your mind to stay present with what is occurring *now*. Yoga consistently questions your assumptions, your view of the world, and ultimately the validity of how you perceive yourself.

Life can feel like a box that constricts and confines. Yoga shows us that whatever box we are trapped within, infinity is with us as well. We have infinite choices, infinite ways to prioritize, infinite things to focus our attention on. As the Buddha said, "We are what we think. All that we are arises with our thoughts. With our thoughts we create the world." By using our mind this way, no matter what the circumstance, we can sense that we are, when all is said and done, infinity in a box.

And we all, saints and sages excluded, have enough dirt on our collars that warrants some neck washing.

The Evolution of EASE

My dream job was turning into a nightmare. I stumbled and lurched at work trying to gain solid footing in the quicksand of reorganizations and a culture that was foreign to me. Feeling that it was important to make a personal contribution to the company in return for a weekly paycheck, I tried to figure out what my role was, exactly. I tried to figure out what was valued by the company.

One barometer I used to see if I was on the right track was the team's monthly report. Like press coverage, the monthly report covers events that would most likely capture the attention of the reader. Writing a brief synopsis of your activities, you could tell what's of interest to the leaders when the condensed report traveled up the chain of command, since each successive level edited the content based on organizational interests.

I noticed that for three months straight, none of my field activities were mentioned in my boss's monthly report to his superior. Not a good sign. So I decided to ask Steve why. His answer, "Because, Megan, your work is not tangible enough."

I wish I could say that I responded with a reasonable approach and asked him to explain and clarify what he meant. It would have been nice to have a professional, grown-up and mature discussion around this topic.

Instead, much to my disgust, I started crying. Not some neat, dainty, slight welling up of the eyes, but a messy, noisy, body-racking, breath-catching embarrassment of uncontrollable sobs. I imagine my boss wished he were having his teeth drilled without anesthesia rather than being on the phone with me at this moment. He spoke quickly, trying to fix the problem by offering solutions. He was trying to fathom how his simple comment had resulted in me losing control.

My inability to work effectively—by my judgment, not others—loomed over me. It all seemed so very important. Work wasn't then, and isn't now, some 9 to 5 thing, a separate piece neatly cleaved off from the rest of my life. Work is an integral expression of me. The comment that my work was "not tangible enough" hit to the core of how I was feeling: invisible.

I was able to hiccup out a request to my boss that day: just give me any specific project that is deemed tangible and valuable to the organization and let that be my responsibility. Just tell me what you want me to do, how you want me to do it, when you need it by and I will spit it out as directed.

I've always preferred creative, new approaches. The colorful, rebel style is more comfortable attire for me than the gray shades of conformity.

My husband has been on the receiving end of my "creativity" early on and on more than one occasion. After returning from our Alaskan honeymoon, I wanted to make him an impromptu special dinner of chicken in white wine. Rummaging through the cupboards, I realized I didn't have all the ingredients. I improvised. As the house permeated with the pungent odor of pickled chicken breast, I realized that there was indeed a difference between white wine and white wine vinegar. My creative side has not always had a desirable outcome.

Perhaps I was trying to make a fancy chicken dinner at work when all that was called for was a burger and fries.

My boss granted my request—giving me specific, measurable tasks that were deemed tangible and valuable to the organization. I had been doing Yoga for a number of years, but it was at this time my Yoga training changed from a physical practice to a mental one.

Since the job did not keep my interest, I played an inner game that is reminiscent of the childhood game "hot/cold." In this game, someone would hide something, and direct another to its spot by saying "hot" or "cold." When you came really close to finding the treasure, you would be "red hot" or "on fire." When you moved further away you were "ice cold."

I paid attention, and became aware of what makes me feel red hot, and what makes me ice cold. Little by little, an inner focus became more central to my day. It's not that my days changed from the way they used to be, but a new awareness was emerging.

The introspective approach I was bringing to work started on the Yoga mat. My teacher would verbally guide the class to feel our body from the inside out, to notice our breathing, to see how our thoughts arose. The same awareness I was cultivating Monday nights from 7:30 to 9:00 in class when executing the Yoga pose "downward dog" came in handy during 9 to 5.

Call it Yoga off the mat.

Everything is Yoga

The sun was shining overhead as a business colleague and I conversed outside work. She was dashing off to another meeting; I was heading back to my office to finish cleaning out my drawers. I had finally quit my job.

She congratulated me, and confided in me the questions she had about her work. These were questions I was familiar with: *Where am I going? What do I want to do with my life? Who am I, really?*

Living with the questions became a spiritual quest for me. Where else does one eventually go for the meaning of life if not to a higher power? At one point I decided to host a small group to discuss spiritual topics. Three of us gathered regularly in my living room, with a fire roaring in the fireplace, and a spread of cheese and crackers with tea laid out before us. It was bound to be interesting; not only were we close friends who loved to celebrate and chat, we also chose to practice our spirituality in ways that were eons apart, at least on the surface. I was a yogi, another was a pagan, and the third was a Catholic. This was not your usual religious roundtable.

One night we were celebrating the eventual end of a New England winter. Although snow was still on the ground, you could smell spring in the air and feel the slightly warmer air on your face. As Ann put another log on the fire, making the already warm room hotter, Jess reached behind to open the window wider. Already the pagan and the Catholic disagreed.

I was stretched out on the sofa enjoying the fact that my two small children were asleep. Quiet rang through the house, something that's entirely too rare for my liking.

Sometimes when we gathered we chose topics to discuss; other times we just followed what came. An unplanned ritual unfolded this evening to fit with the season. We decided to pick a package of seeds that represented what we wanted to plant in our life for the upcoming growing season.

Rummaging through my cupboard, I found a stash of seed packets. I never seem to plant all the seeds that come in an envelope, and for some reason I feel compelled to keep all the half-emptied packets. I stuff them into a box and hide them in a dark corner of the cabinet, which I promptly forget about until after I've bought more seeds for the next planting season. They'll most likely never make it into the ground, but tonight they had a purpose.

Ann, who had made the commitment to show more patience and understanding in her relationship to her husband, appropriately chose the seeds "Sweet Pea." Next, Jess chose the largest seeds from the lot. These would show up in her basket on her altar at home and serve as a reminder of the changing season. I looked through the seed box, wondering which seed packet to pick.

I had made a New Year's resolution a year ago that I was feeling more desperate about. It was not a minor resolution. I wasn't interested in losing ten pounds, exercising more, or eating right, even though I could have benefited from all three. I was only interested in one thing: knowing God. And I wanted to know God experientially, not as some abstract or theoretical construct. Just give me an all-pervasive, all-consuming understanding of the Creator . . . that's all.

My friends knew of this resolution, since I announced it at one of our get-togethers. They understood, then, when I chose the seeds for the flower "Love in a Mist."

It seemed that my concept of God, the intimate contact I craved, was shrouded in a mist. God was there, but I couldn't see clearly. The more I tried to know God, the more aware I became of the void or separation I felt, and the unhappier I became. I suppose the lofty (and some may say impossible) desire to know God was linked to the rather mundane and earthly desire to have satisfying work. I'll bet my paycheck that everyday life and heaven's gate are connected.

On my commute into work one morning, as my mind wondered aimlessly for the 90-minute drive, the proverbial light bulb went off. The punch line was revealed: it's not that Love, or God, is *in* a mist, as the seed package said. Rather, God *is* the mist. There is no place that God is not. Then the void between self and God dissipated. Now that's a good way to begin the day.

I relate this story to you as a prelude to my definition of Yoga. I use the term in its broadest sense—meaning union or wholeness. I do not use the word Yoga to connote only a specific activity, such as breathing exercises or physical postures.

I do use Hatha Yoga (the physical activity most people associate with the term) as a personal practice to know wholeness and union in my everyday life. You may find this wholeness when you're walking outside, hugging your child, or staring into the fire. This book is not about creating converts to a specific school of thought.

Rather, this book advocates a self-directed path to knowing union or wholeness in your own life that does not exclude any aspect of your current reality.

In this book you'll find a smattering of Patanjali's aphorisms (the defining text for classical Yoga) and the Vedic philosophy that serves as the underpinning of the yogic tradition. You're just as likely to find an example of wholeness from the *Harvard Business Review*, a marketing newsletter, or a Buddhist story. You'll find in this text the full spectrum of our twenty-first century life that calls for union.

If wholeness, union, God, emptiness or the divine is omniscient, it's where you are now. If not in this moment, where else would it be? What we're all searching for, the thing that we crave, that we long for in our hearts, is as inseparable as our breath. There simply is no place that it isn't.

The questions my colleague and I were discussing—where am I going, what do I want to do with my life, who am I, really?—were married to the answers. Rainer Maria Rilke answers it best in *Letters to a Young Poet* when he wrote, ". . . .have patience with everything unresolved in your heart and try to love *the questions themselves* as if they were locked rooms or books written in a very foreign tongue. Don't search for the answers, which could not be given to you now, because you would not be able to live them. And the point is, to live everything. *Live* the questions now. Perhaps then, someday far in the future, you will gradually, without even noticing it, live your way into the answer."

With the knowledge that this moment is inherently whole, you can relax. Just trust that where you are now has what you're looking for. This is Yoga.

And with this definition, everything can be Yoga.

∞

What is EASE?

After leaving my job, I decided to share with others the process I had found so helpful. What came from this intention was a four-step approach, called "**EASE**," which combines the introspective techniques of Yoga with the pragmatic demands of everyday life.

EASE is an acronym for a method designed to develop self-knowledge, self-leadership and deliberate living. It's a process to help you see the wholeness of now.

That's right, it's all about you.

Rather than narcissistic self-absorption, self-knowledge is reaching out from the inside with conscious awareness. Most of us run on automatic, trusting that what we know is the truth, and we remain ignorant of our own ignorance. So, the **EASE** process means you make the decision to question everything, including your definition of who you think you are.

Following, in a snapshot, is the process.

Step One: E

E stands for *experience*, the ability to fully connect with the experience you're having in a given moment. Leo Buscaglia sums it up best when he says, "Braille your world," meaning touch, explore and know all there is to know about the moment of now. Life is full of diversity, externally and internally. It's rich with texture, but many times we just skim the surface, not fully experiencing all that's available. When work is frustrating, live that experience fully. When your child gives you a bear hug, live that experience fully. The truth is in the most mundane and the most magnificent daily tasks.

Step Two: A

A stands for *awareness*, the ability we humans have to expand our view beyond our initial limited construct. Just when we feel smug because we have figured something out, we realize there are more layers to uncover. It keeps us humble to know that we don't know. Our hearts stay open and our minds stay young to ask the question "What else is there in this moment?"

Step Three: S

S stands for *self-reflection*. Throughout our lives we ask, "What do I want to do with my life? Where do I want to go? What do I want to get?" This external, future-oriented drive to get, do or be something creates tension. The more pertinent question is *"How do I want to be right now?"* The answer creates a conscious, deliberate path based on the characteristics you wish to express.

Step Four: E2

E2 stands for *elect* or choose. When you have answered the question of how you want to *be*, instead of what you want to *do*, you can experiment with your ability to choose responses that are consistent with your inner values. This is a particularly telling exercise. Actions can frequently be inconsistent with espoused values. Which, of course starts the loop all over again, starting with **E** looking at your experience.

The intrigue of the **EASE** process comes from a personal application to your own life, not from reading. Who wants to just read about flying a plane when you can experience it for yourself? In other words, you are an active participant.

Step One

EXPERIENCE

Braille Your World

Mr. Downey's class was at the top of the stairs on the third floor, the first classroom on the right. I still remember the sound of the junior high school bell summoning the end of one period. The herd of breast-and-pimple-budding adolescents would then migrate in an organized frenzy to the next class. Life was a sharp contrast between friendly, bonding fun and isolating, unsure aloneness.

One day in Mr. Downey's science class, we performed an experiment. In teams of two, one person was blindfolded while the other picked out an object and placed it in an open palm. The blindfolded student wasn't allowed to hold it. Instead, the partner turned the object from side to side against the open palm, until the blindfolded person guessed what the object was: a block of wood. Then the person was allowed to hold it and use all their fingers to explore the block of wood. The truth was quickly discovered: it was a clothespin.

Not being attentive to your life as it's happening is like trying to tell the difference between a block of wood and a clothespin using only the palm of your hand. Too much detail is missing for the truth to be known. From the sketchy outline we jump to conclusions. The underlying assumptions remain hidden. Your experiences become flattened, taking on cookie-cutter sameness. To know the truth we have to explore, touch, and examine the moment we're living.

The first step in the **EASE** process is E for "experience." It's the disciplined ability to examine your own unique experience of the life you're leading.

In a Hatha Yoga class, the teacher instructs you to stay present by noticing different muscles that may be tensing unnecessarily, to notice if your breath is constricted or full, to notice if your mind is scattered or focused. This level of awareness can be practiced in your everyday life as well, outside of Yoga class.

Let me give you a pragmatic example of observing an experience at work as it unfolds.

Think back to a meeting that you found boring. While you were bored, what was your experience? How does boredom affect your breathing? Your energy level? *(I need a nap. . . .)* Your position in the chair? *(Does this back recline any further?)* When you are bored, what thoughts go through your mind? *(I wish he would just stop talking. . . . Maybe I should sit up and nod so it looks like I'm interested. . . . You've got to be kidding. . . .)* What trip does your imagination take? *(I think I'll take the family skiing this weekend. I wonder if the Y has an open racquetball court tonight?)* What actions do you take? *(I'm gonna make a break for the john. . . .)*

Buscaglia's "Braille your world" is a perfect way to sum up the first step of the EASE process. Use all your senses; expand your experience to include the totality of the moment. Notice as much as you can *now* so you don't miss what is going on *now*.

Tuning in does not mean selective reception during only "good" and "desirable" moments. Fully living joy is the same as fully living grief from the perspective of being present with the experience. Both the highs and the lows of life need *you* in order to be fully connected *through* you. You knew this as a young child. One moment you would scream for the candy your mother refused you, the next you giggled with pure joy as you jumped into a pile of leaves. Either way, life was colorful and full of texture. You instinctively brailled your world. You lived in the moment.

In Yoga class, the idea of staying with the difficult as well as the simple postures is called playing with your edge. Finding the point in a posture that's challenging, but not painful for your body, the point where your mind is focused but not stressed, the point where your breath is fully engaged but not constricted, is finding your edge. This limit is where growth occurs. It's the same technique for finding your edges in everyday life: you have to be present to see where your edges are.

You might be questioning the value of staying with such a boring moment, wanting to instead change the experience into something better. This is the "think and grow rich/happy/satisfied" mindset. It's getting out of this moment as it is, and changing it to something that you think suits your needs better that what is being presented. Being in a boring moment is, after all, boring.

Everyone wants peace of mind. Most of us use one of two strategies to obtain it. We either cling tightly to those things we consider enjoyable, wanting to hold onto a good thing, or move away from things we deem distasteful or bad.

The problem with this approach is that it assumes we find peace of mind by perfectly assembling some outside pieces. It assumes that by moving in the direction of external perfection, your inner happiness can shine through. Recently I heard two conflicting messages that go to the heart of the matter.

One message came from a marketing e-newsletter. The suggestion was to steer your work towards being with the type of people you enjoy working with. It makes sense: if you enjoy the people you're working with, the daily tasks and responsibilities can be more enjoyable, and more effective.

The other message was from a Buddhist teacher, who was giving a talk about metta meditation. This meditation is a specific process designed to cultivate loving kindness towards all beings, irrespective of your likes or dislikes. It makes sense: the ability to open your heart to all creates an acceptance of others, making work less stressful, and more effective.

So, do you steer towards work you love, with people you enjoy? Or do you build tolerance and loving kindness in your heart no matter what the circumstance? Let's face it; little details of daily life can be draining.

Since nirvana doesn't seem to be held in finding the perfect job or the perfect person to work with, it's worth cultivating an open heart. It's not to say you shouldn't strive to do work you love with people you enjoy, but don't expect that to be your source of happiness. Fixing the outside environment is not a magic bullet for inner happiness. Spend at least as much time on the inner work as you do on the outer work.

The inner work starts with staying in the present moment. When you think about getting away from a problem, you're living in the future. When you cling tightly hoping that the present won't change, you are living in the past. As you begin the **EASE** process, notice your experience when you're daydreaming about getting a new job because the current circumstances are unbearable. Notice your experience when you're hoping the accolades won't fade, and you think you can't lose.

Here's another reason for staying in the experience of the moment. Staying with the moment means that you notice how you construct your world view. As you practice, you can begin to see how each thought builds upon another, how they come together to form the framework you live within. This is where an inner tug of war begins.

How do I know this meeting is boring? Because I have built this framework of past experiences into this moment. Much of our experience of the world is filtered this way. We hold on to expected norms that dull our ability to actually perceive life on its own terms.

The next time you find yourself in the same old tug-of-war, ask yourself the following question:

What are my thoughts, feelings and actions?

This mental discipline creates a distance from the experience, allowing you to see the experience clearly. It sounds contradictory, but it's not. Have you ever been too close to a problem to see the solution? Perspective is gained by creating space, holding circumstances with an open palm instead of a tight grip. In this way, you're tuning into the observer or witness perspective to gain clarity around your experience.

The observer paradigm is essential to Yoga practice. As you perform postures, the focus is an internal one—noticing thoughts that arise, body sensations that come and go, and the connection to the breath. In Yoga, or for that matter anything we do with mindfulness, we are nourishing and simply noticing what is. By observing, you can begin to see that the label you are putting on your experience is not who you are.

More specific questions may help tease out other aspects of your experience. Questions such as:

> *What emotion is present?*
> *How is my breathing?*
> *What am I saying to myself?*
> *How am I behaving?*
> *What am I feeling in my body?*
> *What is my energy level?*

If you want to begin to see infinity in the box, rather than just the confining walls, notice how the walls are built. Notice everything.

Sitting in a boring meeting, you can answer these questions on a notepad. It will look as if you're taking notes.

You are Sure to Die

Sitting on the back deck late in the summer, I picked up the bubbles my children left behind. Too lazy to return them to the cabinet, I started blowing them into the light breeze. "Too bad they have to go away so fast," said my 91-year-old grandmother as she watched the tiny bubbles float away and then burst.

Life seems to pass just as quickly. I see the truth in the growing faces of my young children and the aged, wrinkled face of my grandmother: everything changes; nothing stays the same. It can be comforting, knowing that bad times will pass. It can be frightening, knowing that the good times will pass as well.

In Yoga class, physical postures can be a way to watch the nature of change within your body. After opening the shoulders in Yoga mudra, for example, an intense muscle experience can change into a flowing movement into the arms and finally end with the realization of a longer and fuller breath.

By watching your own experience closely, you can see the truth of the ever-changing nature of the world. We can all count on one certainty: death. Intellectually we all know that death will come, but today's not the day—there's too much to do. The next day is bad as well. And the next. In fact, death is not part of the plan for the foreseeable future, thank you very much.

Death is a reminder to stay present in the experience of now. A Buddhist nun told me once about a friend who had a car ornament on her dashboard to remind her that death may come at any moment. It was a tiny coffin with a figure dressed in a maroon and yellow robe, looking rather like a nun. Every time the car went over a bump, the little figure would pop up out of the coffin. Rather than a morbid trinket, it was used as a reminder to stay present with life, since it's precious and finite.

There are times when you can feel stuck, as if life is the same struggle day in and day out. That it never changes. Thinking about death can radically change our perception of any circumstance.

You're back at the boring meeting, and you just got an unmistakable message from above: you will die in sixty seconds. No arguments, no time to do anything, just the simple truth that in one minute your life will cease. How would that change your perception of a boring meeting? Would the colors be brighter? Would you see, really see, the people that you worked with? Would you pray for your loved ones?

Looking at your boring meeting from this perspective, you can see how your mind affects your view of the experience. Thinking about death shows how mutable each moment is.

Our experiences are influenced from one moment to the next. That is, one moment of happiness influences positively how the next moment is viewed. Conversely, a problem in one moment negatively affects the subsequent ones. When you argue with your spouse in the morning, it sets the tone at work. Likewise, when you have "a bad day at the office," you're grumpy when you come home.

If moments are habitually classified in the same way, the thoughts create a deep grove in your consciousness, reinforcing a particular thought pattern.

Hence the deep philosophical bumper sticker wisdom, "Same shift, different day."

Most of us don't experience a moment, and then go onto the next in a fresh, unaffected way. Some people hold on for years to wrongs that have been done to them. Others are able to let go of perceived wrongs very quickly. Notice in your own mind and body how one moment effects and builds on the next.

The changing nature of reality can be summed up in the yogic chant "Om." Among other things, Om signifies the transient state of everything in nature. Om is pronounced with three distinct sounds: "Aaaa" "Ooooo" "Mmmm." These three vocalizations correspond to the changing nature of reality. First, comes birth or creation. Then comes sustenance or perseverance. Finally, death or cessation brings the sound to completion.

Om is also the sound of creation, literally. It doesn't *represent* the act of creation that sprang from nothingness. It actually *is* the vibration of creation, the primordial reverberation of existence. In the yogic tradition it's the sound of God; the sound from which the world was created. Om is not unlike the description of the Word in the Book of John that says, "In the beginning was the Word, and the Word was with God, and the Word was God."

Om is the sound that creates everything you see, taste, touch, smell, hear. It creates everything you love, hate, accept, reject. It creates everything you know and everything you don't know. Before, during and after the sound of Om is complete and utter silence. That silence is the wellspring of all creation.

The circle of life happens every moment. Things are born, they live for a while, and then they die. It's simple, predictable and applies to you. The circle of birth through death can be seen in every breath you take, every thought that arises, every body sensation you have.

In the context of the **EASE** process, notice how long you hold on to one moment, even though circumstances have changed. Notice how moments are intertwined. Feel how your interpretation of one moment sets the stage for the next. Once the nature of a thought is seen clearly, you can be the master of it, instead of being its slave.

∞

The Story of Your Life

In his book *Open Minds, Discriminating Minds*, psychologist Charles Tart recounts an experiment conducted at a seminary. The priests in training were asked to give an important sermon across campus. The first group was given ample time to walk over, the second group was told they were late and people were waiting. Along the way, it was arranged that they would come upon a man in obvious need of help. Who would stop to assist?

As you may have guessed, those in the first group, who perceived that they had plenty of time, were more apt to stop and lend a helping hand. Those in the second group, in a hurry to do their duty, were more likely to pass by without helping. The irony is rich since the sermon the priests were hurrying to preach was about the Good Samaritan!

The now you're living is framed by your past experiences that create an understanding of how the world works. You have programmed yourself, by the composite of all your life experiences, to see things the way you think they are. The stories you tell yourself are extremely powerful. They construct a framework for how you interpret your current reality. Therefore, the stories you tell yourself confine possibilities like a box that holds infinity.

The priests were framing their experience in terms of time constraints. How many times have you told yourself that you "never have enough time"?

As you look at your experience, see how you are framing the situation. What are the underlying assumptions you've made about the circumstance?

According to Patanjali, who thousands of years ago compiled a series of "threads" or sutras that stitched yogic philosophy together, there are three components of the mind that create the frames we build. One component records the experience *(Manas)*, another classifies the experience *(Buddhi)* and the last component *(Ahamkar)* relates that experience to your person.

Here's an example of the process of framing from a yogic viewpoint. You see your boss walking quickly down the hall with a red face, as reported by *Manas*. *Buddhi* classifies the information, drawing the conclusion that your boss is angry. *Ahamkar* relates this information to you, making the case that he is mad at you, personally. Based on this framing, you make a decision to take a quick turn into the bathroom!

It should be easy to get a good view of our self. We are, after all, our own best company. As it turns out, clearly seeing our own distortions is a murky business. It begins here in the first step of the **EASE** process, simply noticing your experience, as it is.

What is your experience now as you read these words?

You're Not Too Fat;
Your Pants are Just Too Thin

A visit to my doctor's office usually includes the dreaded event: hopping—lightly I hope—onto the scale for a weigh-in. Bad news: I've gained another five pounds. Life is so unfair. . . .

A typical day can feel like one tug of war after another. Whether we're struggling with weight, the latest reorganization at work, or our children's push for independence, one thing is clear: there would be no tug of war if there weren't another person to play against. No matter how tightly we grasp the rope, how hard we pull, it's just impossible to pull against nothing.

Therefore, when you begin to practice the first step of the **EASE** process, you begin to see that your experience is relational. For example:

- ∞ You're fat and out of shape *in relation* to those irritating height/weight charts in the doctor's office.

- ∞ You're overweight *in relation* to the size of your pants.

∞ You're frustrated *in relation* to your judgment about how things should be.

∞ Your boss is arrogant *in relation* to your past boss.

∞ The vice president is an egomaniac *in relation* to Mother Teresa.

∞ You're mad *in relation* to what you think is "right."

∞ Your spouse is a slob *in relation* to your standards.

Without one, we would have no context with which to place the other. It's the judgment, expectation, and evaluation we place on our experiences. This is what sets up the game of tug-of-war.

As much as it may feel otherwise, your experience is not the absolute truth. The situation is as it is only in context with something else. It helps to use this perspective if you're tired of fighting the tug-of-war. Peace comes when we're ready to let go of being right. In the first step of the **EASE** process, watch how your judgments and expectations create a ripe environment for a tug-of-war.

In Yoga, there is an absolute truth that is independent of comparisons. The Sanskrit term for this truth is *tattva*, meaning that reality which is unchanging, constant and essential. After you begin to see how you're setting up the relational tug-of-war, you're in a stronger position to control it in a positive way, and reside in the larger truth.

If you're not the sole keeper of truth, it allows for possibilities. Your boring meeting is boring compared to skydiving. But it's positively adventurous compared to watching paint dry.

∞

It Is As It Is

There's one more important thing about how you perceive your experience: it's valid. Your perspective is real and tangible. How you feel, how you interpret a given moment is just that— how you see it. You do not need to continue the cycle and judge your judgments. That would be a never-ending hell.

The point of watching and observing your experience is so you know it for what it is. It is a way of honoring all yourself, not just the parts you think are right, moral or good. It's is also a way of honoring others. How others perceive the world is just that— how they see it.

With this in mind you have set the stage for the next step in the **EASE** process.

Summary

- Notice everything about your life experience. Delve into the moment by asking yourself: what are my thoughts, feelings and actions?

- Your experience, like everything else, changes. It's not a static thing.

- Your experience is framed by the stories you tell yourself. Listen to the voices in your head, noticing how they construct the drama.

- Your experiences are relational. Yours is not the absolute truth.

- Your experiences are valid. Honor them.

Step Two

Awareness

Less Than 1%

In *Emotional Alchemy, How the Mind can Heal the Heart*, author and psychotherapist Tara Bennett-Goleman shares a startling statistic: less than one percent of the information our mind takes in actually reaches our awareness. That means 99% of our experience is filtered out as if we never lived it.

The next step in the **EASE** process is **A**, which stands for awareness. This is the ability we have to broaden our perspective in a given moment.

Here's an exercise for you to do right now. Take your attention to your big toe. Notice where it is and how it feels. Is it hot or cold? How does your sock feel against your toe? Can you feel your shoe pushing against it? Which toe are you examining, the right or left? Can you feel the contact with the adjoining toe?

A moment ago, you were probably oblivious to your big toe. The simple act of bringing your attention to it, however, has expanded your current experience to include the sensation of your toe.

When you have a problem, your attention goes to that, effectively screening out other input. In the next step of the **EASE** process, after you've given the experience a thorough exploration, you can then expand your awareness to include other possibilities. The relationship between your experience and your awareness is:

- ∞ Your Experience is the window frame. Your Awareness is the view out the window.

- ∞ Your Experience is the concept these words are conveying. Your Awareness is the space between the words.

- ∞ Your Experience answers the question "What am I thinking and feeling?" Your Awareness answers the question "What else is there?"

Webster's *New World Dictionary* defines "awareness" as: "knowing or realizing; conscious; informed." Personally, I like the concept of "realizing" as a way of describing awareness. It suggests that a new understanding has been uncovered.

Awareness is a continuum. The broadening of awareness might simply mean seeing a situation through a new framework in your own mind. Broadening your awareness may mean seeing the problem from another's perspective, or seeing the problem from a system's perspective or perhaps in relation to the world at large. On the furthest end of the awareness continuum is the perspective of universal consciousness.

In Yoga, connecting with this universal perspective is called *samadhi*, a state of being where your well-known borders of self dissolve into pure awareness. *Samadhi* is where your labels of self cease to be, and instead you simply rest in pure being. Written or verbal accounts of this state always describe it as a grand, unimaginable bliss. The problem with this description is that the mind then tries to frame the description of what "bliss" must feel like. By doing this comparison, we're setting ourselves up for the tug-of-war, undermining the power of our own experience. Looking for *samadhi* keeps us reaching for something in the future, as if it were a goal that needed to be reached. Let's keep it simple and imagine that we all have experienced *samadhi*. It's the still spot between the in-breath and the out-breath. It's the simple contentment of holding your baby's hand. It's the pure heaven of a tired body in a warm bed. It's just resting in the moment and releasing the sense of "me." Forget about the grandiose words describing *samadhi*, and instead find it in this moment.

Practicing awareness creates space so that you can stop your automatic reaction mode. Reactions happen internally first, at the speed of thought, and then go out externally through the action of words or behavior.

The first aspect of expanding our awareness is the desire or intention to look at the problem in a new context. That's all, just a willingness to open and explore other possibilities. This is easier said than done. Sometimes we're so caught up in being right, or being angry, that we don't want to consider other possibilities. We want to stay as mad and as righteous as we are now. If this is how it is for you, step away from the antagonizing situation or person to limit harm, and continue to be present to your experience. Stay with the experience. Sooner or later it will change.

The next aspect that's helpful for expanding awareness is to relax. Softening the edges, letting go of your grip on the rope slightly, even if it is only in a minuscule way. From my experience, this typically means slowing down or stepping away from the problem.

∞

Easier Said Than Done

Words are easy to write. Actions can be trickier.

There are always those in life who see things differently. I worked with a man once who was my opposite. I said black; he said white. He said up, I said down. We saw the world from diametrically opposed views. Part of it was our assigned roles and responsibilities within the organization: he managed a customer segment that was in constant conflict with my segment. The field issues and turf battles bubbled up to us, and we each tended to view the problem from our constituent's perspective.

Not only were we on different wavelengths from an organizational perspective, we were also on a different wavelength personally. Sometimes a relationship just clicks. Sometimes it doesn't. We were far from clicking.

Like it or not, to complete an assigned project we needed to work together, and found ourselves in a series of ongoing meetings. Sitting across from one another, it would take all of five minutes before the first dividing issue came up. With each progressive meeting my tolerance for this man would diminish. At the next meeting, when it only took two minutes for the dividing issue to smack the middle of the table, I watched myself.

My experience consisted of anger. Frustration. Mentally rolling my eyes. Breathing quickly. Temperature rising. Narrowing of focus. Incoherent thoughts.

I realized that his mouth was moving, but my brain was not registering what was being said. Remember Charlie Brown's teacher who just says "Blah, blah, blah, blah . . . "? That was what I was hearing. I sternly yelled at myself: LISTEN!

And you know what happened? Nothing. I still couldn't hear what he had to say. And he still bugged me.

Sometimes when we try to gain some space from a situation, to get clarity and increase our awareness in the moment, we can't. Sometimes the most we can do is ride the roller coaster of our experience.

Another story with a different ending came from New York City. I had completed my work early, so I was at LaGuardia Airport long before my flight was due to depart. LaGuardia is a hectic airport, especially in the shuttle area where I was waiting. Every few minutes a new flight would be boarded, the lines to the counter were long, and there was a shortage of seats. This was barely controlled chaos.

Having finally made it to the counter, I handed my ticket to the agent and overheard the person next to me ask for help. She was a young woman whose name I don't remember. I do, however, remember the name of her dog: Ginger. The name aptly described her—her coat was the color of ginger spice, and she had a warm, kind disposition that makes you think of gingerbread baking. Perhaps this is why I am able to recall the dog's name and not her master's.

Ginger was a seeing-eye dog who needed to go to the bathroom before she embarked on her journey to Maine, and the pair needed an escort outside. I volunteered. Guiding them through the long walk from shuttle area to the outside world, it became clear how much I use visual clues for communicating. To a blind person, the directions "It's just over here" or "this way" aren't in the least bit helpful. A simple "right" or "left" will suffice.

We successfully made it outside, more on the merit of Ginger following my moves than the owner following my awkward verbal directions. Outside of LaGuardia the smells assaulted me. Did you ever notice how all big-city airports are made the same? You exit the baggage area and end up trapped in a tunnel-like roadway congested with vehicles picking up passengers. It's like breathing in the exhaust from an unventilated auto body shop. I was just about to make a wise comment about the fresh air, when the owner said, "I can smell the grass." I laughed, thinking she had made a joke. "You're kidding, right?" I asked. No, she swore she could smell the little postage-size patch of green weeds off to our right.

Now that's a great example of expanding awareness. If someone can smell grass at LaGuardia's arrival station, then we certainly have a fighting chance to smell roses in the thorn of our problem.

Yes, expanding our awareness is easier said than done. Yet forcing the issue does nothing. In fact, the opposite is true. Relaxing with the current reality is the path to release and eventual expansion of awareness.

What is Awareness?

Awareness holds infinite possibilities.

In the E step, you explored how you framed the world, how the boundaries were constructed. Expanding awareness is the ability to look beyond our construct and entertain the idea that there are possibilities other than the one we have accepted as "right." Awareness, at the far end of the spectrum, is non-relational.

In order to judge something, one thing had to be compared to something else. Awareness, on the other hand, is non-relational. That is, things just are they way they are, without regard for how they compare to another. Awareness is, at its core, the ability to hold diametrically opposed information as a whole.

During a nuclear physics class I took in college, we studied the characteristics of subatomic particles. A photon, or packet of energy, was an interesting thingamajig in this tiny, unseen world. This "packet of energy" confounded scientists for the longest time. Confounded them because they couldn't decide whether it was a particle (had mass) or a wave (had energy). The photon seemed to be both of these things at once.

Experiments showed that at times this photon took on properties of a particle, at times it was a wave. Most interesting of all was the fact that the observer, the so-called impartial witness, had a bearing on the results. The photon was neither a particle nor a wave. The photon was both a particle and a wave. The scientific uproar that followed this discovery was monumental. There was no conventional resolution. Instead, the scientists learned to live with the paradox that this thingamajig was both a particle and a wave. And it was neither a particle nor a wave. This grand dichotomy opened the doors to a whole new and exotic way of viewing the world of subatomic particles.

The larger you expand your awareness, the more apt you are to see conflict as a whole, rather than as singular parts. When you do this with your individual issues, you can hold the conflicts more lightly; you can eventually let go of the rope. The tug-of-war seems less intense if you can watch your mind settle on the whole of two sides of a coin rather than choose one or another.

Could infinity fit in a box?

Awareness and Your Intention

Awareness involves an intention of focus. Some would use the word discipline, but I have found that that definition sets up an internal force or pressure to make some things happen. No need to add to tension, so use the word intention instead.

Webster's *New World Dictionary* defines intention as: "1. a determination to act in a specified way or 2. purpose." In order to see beyond and deeper into our experience, there must be some internal motivation, some purpose for doing so. What is your purpose or reasoning for wanting to look at a larger perspective? There are many valid reasons. Perhaps you're just plain tired of running the same scenario over and over again in your mind. Perhaps you're sick of complaining about a problem. Perhaps you're just curious about what else is in this thorny issue. Perhaps you're bored. Whatever the reason, it's helpful to explore your motivation for expanding your awareness. A clear purpose or determination will help you stick with the work this introspective approach takes.

What benefits would you gain if you expanded your awareness?

Awareness is Real

A broader awareness is just as valid as your experience. That is, expanding your awareness does not invalidate your personal experience. Both have their place. Take, for example, being mugged. If you've been attacked on the street I'm doubtful that you took the opportunity, consciously at least, to explore and expand your awareness in that moment. Instead, we react to protect ourselves the best we can.

At times it can seem as if we are trapped in a constrictive circumstance. There is no sense that a larger awareness exists, since our everyday experience is one of difficulty and struggle. During such periods it feels as though the universe is conspiring against us, with circumstances driving an incessant, relentless march towards an inevitable confrontation. Whether it's getting out of an abusive or lifeless relationship, stepping off the corporate roller coaster, or saying good-bye to a friend who has been fighting a long war with illness, the seeds of the situation have been have been long planted.

When circumstances feel inevitable, seemingly beyond our control, what keeps us from a downward spiral? If we are drowned by the enormity of our experience, unable to expand our awareness, what can we hold on to for comfort? For me, the answer is trust.

There's a Yoga saying that states, "That is perfect, this is perfect. What comes from such perfection truly is perfect. What remains after perfection from perfection is yet perfect." That's a whole lot of perfection for an apparently imperfect world.

Since imperfection seems to be everywhere, it takes trust to believe in perfection. When times are tough, where do you place your trust? Do you trust your own wisdom? Do you trust the support of loved ones? Do you trust some unseen, greater force? Placing your trust in something you believe in is an acknowledgment that there is a greater awareness than your experience would believe. Through trust, awareness is expanded instead of contracted.

Whether it's the pain of war that forces us to see the need for peace, or the pain of death that shows us the value of life, trust can be something to hold onto until the calmer waters of peace are reached.

Be an Observer

Have you ever watched the show *Candid Camera*? As you observe the participant's reaction to the stunt being performed, it's easy to see how they are framing and reacting to their experience. Some people react incredulously, some in anger, some in panic. As I giggle at the responses, a part of me is glad *I* wasn't exposed to the joke, since I might embarrass myself. We can look more objectively at the situation because we're observing it rather than identifying with it. Sometimes it even seems unbelievable that a person sees this setup as a plausible event. Again, we have the perspective of an observer, not as an active participant. This gives us an advantage.

You can see the candid camera dynamic in business meetings. Two people have opposing views. As you sit in the meeting, you're able to watch these two bang heads. Even if you try to intervene, it's to no avail. They are caught up in their view of the world, and are unable to open up to possibilities. Being an observer is easy when you are the third party.

Working with the **A** step, the idea is to observe *yourself*, so you're able to see more broadly. This is easiest to do when you are quiet or restful. Initially, it's most difficult to do when you're agitated or upset. So the trick is to practice the art of self-observation when you're not stressed-out. This leads us to the next activity to expand awareness.

∞

Breathe

Since we breathe so much, you'd think we'd have it down pat. But breathing is so automatic we tend to overlook it as a way to slow us down in order to increase awareness. In an automatic mode, breathing tends to get shallow when we're stressed, short when we're angry, and tight when we're frustrated. When we're relaxed and calm our breathing is longer, fuller and deeper. There's a close connection between how you're breathing and your emotional state. Thus, it's a great tool when you are feeling overwhelmed by emotion.

The next time you have a million things to do, and the boss needs the report *now,* and your computer chooses today to go on the blink, breathe. Take a moment or two to take long, deep, full, complete breaths. The more you do this exercise, the more it works. If you find it difficult to slow down your breathing, take a short walk. Let the fresh air open your lungs. After the walk notice how your breathing has changed.

The core of any Yoga practice is breathing, or *pranayama*. *Prana* is a Sanskrit word meaning life or life energy. *Ayama* means extension. Thus *pranayama* is an extension of life energy. Breath is the external manifestation of this invisible life force. With each inhale and exhale, life energy flows in and out of our body. Gain mastery over the breath, and you gain control of life energy.

There are many ways to work with this life energy through breathing techniques.

One simple technique is to just watch your breath as it comes in and out of your body. You breathe all day, now do it with conscious awareness. The mere act of focusing on your breathing will center and calm your mind.

Another technique is a variation of alternate nostril breathing in Yoga. While sitting comfortably, imagine you are breathing up the left side of your body, pulling air in through the sole of your left foot. Trace the left side of your body in your mind in great detail until you reach the top of your head at the peak of your inhalation. Then exhale, tracing in your mind's eye the right side of your body as carefully as you did the left. Finish this one breath cycle by exhaling through the sole of your right foot. On the next breath, reverse the process and inhale through the right sole of your foot, up to the top of your head, and exhale through the left foot. Continue this pattern and end by breathing out through the right foot. The purpose of this exercise is to help balance and create harmony.

Another breathing exercise helps increase the fullness of your breathing and concentrate your mind. It's called three-part yogic breathing. You can do this sitting, standing or lying down. Simply inhale deep into the abdomen, then take that same breath into your middle chest, and then continue that same breath into your upper chest, to the space right under your shoulders. Then exhale from the abdomen, middle chest, and then upper chest. Continue this rhythm of full, complete, even breaths, opening your body and relaxing your mind.

There are hundreds of breathing techniques. Your best bet is to just start noticing how your breathing affects your thought patterns and vice-versa. You'll be amazed how simple and effective breath awareness is for modulating the mind.

Go to the Library

We tend to gravitate towards the same type of information. Whether it's for work or for pleasure, the more diverse our information, the broader our perspectives can be. The library is a treasure trove for expanding awareness. During your lunch break, or in between sales calls while you're on the road, visit a library. Don't go with a particular book in mind. Instead, just allow yourself to meander through the stacks, your eyes scanning the titles. See where you end up. Intentionally pick up something that's different for you to read, outside of your everyday topics.

Interestingly enough, I've found that when I have an interest or a problem on my mind, no matter what book I choose, it will have some relevance. This interconnectedness fascinates me. Expanding your awareness is not a linear, black and white process. Rather, it is more like a bowl of messy spaghetti with the strands twisted and connected in impossible ways.

∞

Change a Pattern

On this same subject of interconnectedness, we can open our awareness by changing any pattern, not necessarily one associated with a problem.

Jean Houston speaks and works widely on creativity and expanding connections in our minds. One exercise she talks about reminds me of a childhood game that was always good for a laugh.

First, you start by patting your head. Next, while still patting your head, you begin to rub your abdomen. While you keep all this up, you begin to hop on one foot. Then maybe start singing. It's quite silly, but according to Houston it helps break old patterns and enables you to see new perspectives. You can do this in the office if you like, although I suspect it might be noted in your personnel records.

Breaking patterns can be small, like getting up on the opposite side of the bed. Or listening to country music instead of talk radio. Or taking a different route to work. Or taking Yoga instead of kickboxing.

Perhaps your morning in the office looks something like this: turn on office lights, boot up the computer, listen to voice mail, check the schedule, go to the bathroom, get a cup of coffee. Most likely you do these things in the same order every day. Such was the case for a group of healthcare administrators at an annual conference in Las Vegas, where I was giving a presentation. While talking about the power of habits, I suggested that they make a change in their morning routine. Consider, for example, a cup of tea instead of coffee. The audience groaned. Take a different way in to work then. More groans. They didn't seem particularly enamored with the ideas.

Most of us are married to our current habits. There's nothing inherently wrong with our morning routine, but if we can get accustomed to new approaches with something manageable—like tea instead of coffee—it can strengthen our ability to be flexible when the stakes are higher—like a reorganization at work.

Doing little things like taking a new way into work may seem trivial. It may even seem like more mental work than is necessary for a brain already consumed with the many tasks the day ahead holds. In fact, experimentation with new, little things helps the mind become more flexible with the bigger problems. And with the big problems, having an open and flexible mind can be a lifesaver. As Albert Einstein said, "Problems cannot be solved at the same level of awareness that created them."

When we put our bodies into new and different positions, like the unique Yoga postures, we are changing routines. Consider the way you're sitting while reading this book. Is it the same position you assume while working on the typewriter? Examine the way the body is positioned the next time you're waiting in line at the grocery store or having a conversation with a friend. Do you tend to shift one hip out? Favor the weight in one leg over another? Body habits, just like habits of the mind, are built up over time. Just like a car needs a tune-up, our bodies can use some realignment over time. Doing a headstand may not be your cup of tea, but it certainly changes your perspective and view of the world.

Think Circular, Not Linear

In the *Harvard Business Review* article, "The Making of a Corporate Athlete," (Jan. 2001) authors Jim Loehr and Tony Schwartz draw an analogy between top-ranking athletic training and the work of corporate executives. One point they make is that athletes build periods of rest and recovery into their training in order to optimize performance and growth from "work-out" time. Executives, on the other hand, tend to push longer and harder in order to make things happen. Time away from work can be seen as "wasted."

Loehr and Schwartz make the case that it is during such "down" time that real progress can be made. Termed "mental oscillation," taking a break and doing something that does not involve cognitive functions can increase your mental capacity. It seems that having a facial, massage, or game of golf in the afternoon is not such a bad idea. No need, then, for guilt.

Our Newtonian, linear, cause-and-effect culture highly values a no-nonsense approach to work and work ethics. Your personal experience tells you that when you have a break you are fresher and more able to handle stress. It is not the stress itself that does you in; it is the inability to recuperate sufficiently to continue. As Loehr and Schwartz point out in the Harvard Business Review article, most of us work at a sprinter's pace for the duration of a marathon.

Yoga students notice interesting nonlinear connections during the course of class. The man who complains of neck problems notices relief when the hips are opened and stretched. The woman who has been having migraines notices they go away if she includes breathing exercises into her daily routine. The body is a beautiful example of an interconnected web.

Instead of a linear pattern of thinking, allow meandering, seemingly unrelated activities to enter your day.

Because, as it turns out, everything is related.

∞

See Your Labels

The first time I attended a class at Insight Meditation Center in Barre, Massachusetts, I didn't know what to expect, so I scoped out the room before I entered. Cushions and chairs were laid out in a circle on a maple floor so polished and smooth you could skate across it. People sat as still and quiet as statues in different positions. All had their eyes closed.

Walking across the floor in my socked feet, I decided to sit on a cushion. Sitting cross-legged seemed so meditative. I snuck a peek at my watch, and it said 6:00 P.M. I was right on time. I waited for the class to begin. I closed my eyes and waited some more. I waited and waited. My back groaned and my mind wrestled with nothing. The open windows to summer called. Finally, I could stand it no longer. No matter how meditative that crossed-legged position looked, I was moving up to the chair. I snuck another peek at my watch: 6:30. Obviously the class had already started. Is this what we do for a whole hour? I squirmed and squiggled, trying to get comfortable. Can't we meditate lying down?

Finally, the leader spoke. I now had something else to focus on besides my aching back. Buddha, the leader said, teaches us that when an enlightened person meets someone, they're not seen as either superior or inferior. A smug little voice in my head finished the Buddha's lesson by boastfully saying, "Of course, we are all equals." My mind was self-satisfied with its conclusion.

Only the leader didn't finish the story in this way. Instead, he said the Buddha teaches us that an enlightened person does not see others as superior, inferior, OR EQUAL. My mind was caught off guard, and spent the rest of the meditation searching for understanding.

In most cases, when we're describing who we are, we answer with roles and responsibilities. I'm a mother. I'm an account executive. A salesperson. A musician. An artist. That's not who you are; that's your job title. It's a handy label that boxes you into some framework that the other person can relate to. Don't ever confuse what you do with who you are. You're much too grand to fit into a puny label.

Try this one on for size: you are that you are. If we must choose a label, let's make it big, really big. Let's just say: I am. A friend of mine who used to be a nun told me that this was how God described himself. I AM THAT I AM.

Descartes said, "I think, therefore I am." Or perhaps he said it in a more philosophically eloquent way, "I think, ergo I am." Well, here's a new rendition, "I am, therefore I am." I am that I am; others are that they are. There is no superior, no inferior, no equal. It just is that it is.

There is a yogic mantra that represents this same view. It's the *Hamsa* (or *So'ham*) mantra. A mantra, by the way, is simply a sound that when repeated has the power to transform consciousness. It's said that the *Hamsa* mantra is the natural mantra of an individual, flowing with each breath in and out of the body.

The first syllable, *Ham,* is created by the in-breath and starts the creative process of your self. It is the birth of "I" from the divine source. When you exhale, the sound of *sa* is the absorption of that moment of self back to its source. It's the death of "I." The natural silence after each exhalation is absolute awareness, divine dissolution of self into source. In English, the rough translation of *Hamsa* is "I am that." By repeating the mantra, you begin to identify that which you call "I" as something much grander than mundane labels.

You are neither the labels given to you nor the roles you have played, whether you have assumed them willingly or not.

You don't have to believe me on this one (or any point for that matter). Check it out for yourself. If repeating the *Hamsa* mantra isn't for you (although I recommend you give it a try) here's another option. Write out a list of ten words that describe the type of person you are (caring, loving, patient, impatient, mean, etc.). Don't spend a lot of time on it, just jot them down as they come to you. After you've done this, go through the list one by one and ask yourself, "When haven't I been this quality?" You'll see that you're none of the qualities all of the time.

The second way to do this exercise is write a list of words that describe your nemesis, or at least someone you disagree with. Quickly list ten qualities that come to mind about this person. After you're done, go through the list and ask, "Have I ever displayed these qualities?" If you look deeply and honestly, perhaps you can say yes. We're all human, and we can hold the full spectrum of human potential from the most dangerous to the most exalted. It may be only a matter of degrees, but looking deeply, we can touch upon each piece in our own heart.

Doing this exercise can also spark the question, "If I'm not these things all the time, who essentially am I?"

∞

If You Think You're Right, Write

At times, we don't see eye-to-eye with another. The more emotionally charged the topic is, the more difficult it is to see the situation clearly. This lesson became clear to me while on business in Pittsburgh.

While having breakfast with my boss, I slid as gracefully as I could into the vinyl-upholstered bench that never fails to create static cling. As I sunk into the soft cushion, my boss sat across from me in the chair, giving him the height advantage. I tried to sit tall.

I glanced at the menu. Eating breakfast in hotels so often, I knew the typical menu and what I would order.

Dan and I discussed the upcoming meeting I'd coordinated and would lead later that morning. After dispensing with the meeting details, I asked him if I could attend an organizational dynamics conference. His response caught me completely off guard.

Dan looked at me and said, "Megan, it seems that all this reading and learning is separating you from the group." He proceeded to tell me how my vocabulary and way of viewing the world was not in sync with others, and they had a hard time understanding me. Going to another conference would not help. He also added that when I stood up in front of a group to make a point, rather than staying seated in my chair, it alienated people. "Grandstanding" is the term he used (at least it's the term *I* remember).

Later that morning, I led the team meeting with my bottom firmly rooted in the safety of my chair. The feedback had rocked my world. I no longer knew how to conduct myself in a meeting in a way that would be acceptable to the group. I chose to be quiet.

This was difficult information to process. Back in my hotel room after the meeting, I could finally spend some time working with it. I got mad. I felt an injustice had been done. I thought I would get my resume together. Then I called a good friend to discuss it and got very sad.

Feeling alienated from the work group, struggling to find a place, I started to write in my journal. In the process of writing, I found healing. In some odd way, the act of writing can reveal things that lay hidden. Writing creates a new view.

Here are two exercises to try when you're feeling hurt.

The first exercise involves answering three simple questions. The first question is "What is the truth of that which I'm finding most difficult to accept?" The remark that I was grandstanding was painful to hear. Was there truth in this remark? OK, I am a bit of a ham, so the term "grandstanding" is not completely off the mark. When people hurt you with words, is there a grain of truth in it for you to own? Write down all that comes to mind.

The second question to ask yourself concerning the truth of the matter is to examine why you did it. For me, grandstanding for ego gratification was only part of why I behaved as I did. I also had a strong desire to move the group forward, to help clarify and communicate concepts using a flip chart. Asking yourself "Why do I do this?" gets to the heart of your own motivation for your behavior. Write down in your journal all that comes to mind.

The third question to explore is "How can I modify my behavior to be true to myself and respectful of others?" In my case, I decided to stand less, and listen more. I was surprised by the results: I learned more from others and found I didn't have the only answer to problems.

To summarize the first writing exercise, write the answer to these three questions:

> *Is there a grain of truth in what this person is saying?*
> *Why do I behave this way?*
> *How else could I behave?*

This second exercise may be helpful if you can't find any grain of truth in what the person has done or said.

Take a situation where you had a "confrontation" or a strong disagreement. The confrontation comes from your thoughts, if not your actions or words. It's not necessary for heated words to be exchanged, but you do have a strong opposition about it as measured by the tightening of your gut and the thoughts in your mind. This tug-of-war is serious.

Later, spend some time writing a short story reviewing the scene. It's not for others, so feel free to just let it out. This part of the exercise is completely from your perspective, not from your opponent's.

Now comes the fun part. Take the same situation and write it from the perspective of the other person. Do this with one caveat:

pretend that the person felt right, justified or at least not wrong in the actions or thoughts they displayed. Obviously, this is a guessing game. It's hard enough to get to the truth of our own mind, much less the mind of another.

The purpose of the exercise is to help you soften or relax what you're holding on to. It's not to say you won't still feel right or justified in your view, but perhaps it helps you see a paradox: that you're right, and the other person may not be wrong. This is the beginning of redefining the rules of the tug-of-war game.

I did this exercise with the breakfast meeting I had with my boss, Dan. Writing from my perspective I could better understand my motives for standing up in front of a group. Personally, I have found that there's a correlation between the amount of hurt or defensiveness a comment causes and the value of the truth that can be found when exploring it. Defensiveness or hurt can be seen as a signal indicating the need for personal exploration.

For example, I found it painful when I was told that getting up in front of the group was "grandstanding" and that my actions were separating me from others. Looking deeper, I saw that I identified myself with the label of a "good communicator." I was proud of this skill. I also realized that standing up to make my point was partly ego driven. As I said, there is a ham in me that loves to be the center of attention. Doing the writing exercise, I could see those parts of myself more clearly, and then more objectively see the impact these behaviors had on the group.

Writing from Dan's perspective, I could play with the possibility that he was trying to help. His feedback could help me fit into the group better and be accepted. In his mind, he was being caring. He was doing what managers do: providing important and constructive feedback—even if it's difficult to give—for the purpose of professional development and growth. Of course this perspective may be wrong, but it really doesn't matter. I'm not trying to define Dan; I'm trying to soften my hold on the rope.

Whether we agree or not, another's actions are right or justified from their view of the world. This is hard to swallow if we're vehemently opposed to the actions or view of another. But the truth is most people don't do anything that's warped or wrong from their inner construct of the world. They might label it as wrong in retrospect, when after the fact it's seen as inappropriate. However, in the moment of action, it was the right thing to do; otherwise it wouldn't have been done. Given a certain framework of reality, in a given time, any action can seem "right" in the eye of the beholder. Or, at the very least, it doesn't seem wrong.

Seeing a situation from another's view can be eye opening, even disturbing. This is why it's a great way to open your awareness.

The Left/Right Column Exercise

Earlier, I alluded to the fact that I was feeling impotent at work. A rather nasty word but one that aptly describes my experience. No matter how hard I tried, I was unable to make a contribution that seemed worthwhile to me or was viewed as tangible by the organization. What I noticed by staying with my experience was that during team meetings my mental state fluctuated between agitation *(here we go again with another strategic plan that will go nowhere...)* and hopelessness *(what a waste of time...)*. My interaction within the group echoed these inner thoughts. I either said nothing or was outwardly opposed to the process. And neither was very helpful for me or for the group dynamics.

One day while commuting to work, I thought about the upcoming meeting. How could I be more productive? I decided to only say something if it helped the group process along. Predictably, the same issues were discussed, and I saw the same thoughts running through my mind. "Only add to the group discussion in a productive manner," I reminded myself. I didn't say much at that meeting. Even when a co-worker snapped at me, I had no retort. Stay productive, I told myself.

This did not work for expanding my awareness. All it did was lock up my frustration.

I knew I needed help, so I decided to do something I had never done before: I hired a consultant. I had worked with plenty of consultants before for business-related projects, but had never hired one personally just for a problem I was having.

I was fortunate enough to come across a wonderful woman who specialized in Organizational Development, and she helped me uncover assumptions that made an impact on my subsequent behavior. One exercise I did while working with her was the left/right column exercise. Here's how it works.

Take a piece of paper and draw a line down the middle. On the left side of the paper, write the comments that were going through your head when you had an interaction that frustrated you. On the right side of the column write everything that was said in a given time frame. Obviously, you wouldn't write out a whole hour's worth of conversation from your memory, so choose just those moments that were the most frustrating and stick out in your mind.

As you see what thoughts were coming up, and you notice the corresponding words you spoke, ask yourself the following questions:

Was what I was thinking versus what I was saying?

How do these unspoken thoughts affect my behavior?

What do these thoughts imply about my assumptions?

Why didn't I say what was on my mind?

When I completed this exercise my underlying assumptions were clear: I thought I was right. The mere concept that I was right meant, in the tug-of-war game, that others were wrong. My behavior, therefore, was confrontational even though I thought I was being accommodating.

Look at the thoughts you wrote on the left hand side of the paper. Examine the words you spoke on the right hand side of the paper. What does the difference between the two say about your underlying assumptions?

There is a saying in Yoga: as in your practice, so too in life. If a person tends to fight and force Yoga postures, then this pattern will be seen in everyday situations. If a person consistently gives up on postures prematurely, this pattern will be seen in life as well. Whether you're studying Yoga or a new database at work, your underlying assumptions about the world can be ferreted out if you stay aware and alert.

Play the "What If. . . ." Game

Have you ever had a spectacular failure at work or in life? I have. And it can make a person crave anonymity.

After I left the security of a weekly paycheck, I thought I was going to "wow" audiences with a thought-provoking and original seminar designed to create inner calm in a chaotic and crazy corporate world. I was so sure that this topic was a hit that I remember asking the hotel sales coordinator if I could expand the meeting space if I had too many registrants. "Of course," she said. "This ballroom can hold up to three hundred and fifty people."

I ended up moving to a small cubicle of a room that I filled with family and friends, ten in all.

When you're unable to expand your awareness in the heat of the moment, and circumstances don't match your expectations, there are two things that can help you move on. The first is to see your expectations clearly. The second is to play the "What if. . . ." game.

Your expectations set the gauge for judging success or failure. What is success except a measurement in relation to your expectation? So, if you had a grand failure, chances are you had a grand expectation. Good for you.

How tedious it would be to live with only "realistic" expectations. Continue to think grand. As Nietzsche said, "Life is a thousand times too short for us to bore ourselves."

Do see clearly, though, the divergence between your expectation and the current reality. This is where the "What if. . . ." game comes in handy. It can refocus your awareness by modifying your approach rather than limiting your expectations.

So, in the case of your spectacular failure, ask yourself:

"What if I did this . . . ?"
"What if I did that . . . ?"
"What if I changed this . . . ?"

This mental game helps build a flexible mind—a mind willing to experiment and to explore. It also takes the focus off of the constricted feeling of failure and opens up new possibilities to consider. The "what if" game builds a valuable learning bridge between actions and results.

When a problem arises, stay with your experience. Later, when you have some distance from it, do the left/right column exercise. See if it uncovers your underlying assumptions. These assumptions, by the way, are fairly obvious once they are unveiled. Intellectually you will say "Of course." Emotionally, however, these assumptions will resonate in a way that affects your immediate experience. You know the assumptions are the ones for you to work with if you feel an inner shift, like a click-into-place of a realization. If you don't feel, see or sense it, don't worry.

Stay with your experience and put the exercise away for the time being. Come back to it tomorrow. And the next day. Sooner or later you will see how your foundation is created.

Once you have seen the concept you are functioning under, play the "What if. . . ." game. *What if* I didn't hold this belief? *What if* there were another alternative? *What if* . . . .

You can even play the "What if. . . ." game with Yoga. Many times we see the teacher or guru as being the ultimate authority. Question authority by testing the instructions against your own experience. Play with the "correct" alignment to see if it's correct for your body. External measurements of perfection are not the point of Yoga; inner awareness is.

Whether it's in Yoga class or at a staff meeting, see how playing "What if. . . ." changes both your perception and your behavior. See how the "What if. . . ." game opens your awareness. There's wisdom to be gained by incorporating learning feedback loops into your activities, no matter what the outcome.

We seldom question success. What if . . . you did?

Summary

- Explore options and possibilities in your life by asking yourself: what else is there in this moment or situation?

- There is always more to your experience than can ever be taken in by your senses. Awareness holds infinite possibilities.

- When you are ready and willing to broaden your perspective, focus on cultivating your observer paradigm. Practice being the witness of the moment.

- Focus on your breath to relax your body and train your mind.

- Try new things to expand your mind. Go to the library, take a different route to work, intertwine rest and recovery periods into your busy life, and try writing to uncover your hidden assumptions about the world.

- Your awareness is non-relational; it's always there no matter what the circumstances. Full and complete awareness is the absolute truth.

- Expanding your awareness is valid. Honor the fact that there are other options even if you're unable to see them.

Step Three

SELF REFLECTION

What Do You Want to Be When You Grow Up?

I was upstairs in the loft tickling my four-year-old daughter. The sun shone through the skylight as Emily's little-girl giggles permeated the house. Just the sound of it made me laugh. She was playing baby, curling up in a small handmade crib that my mother had made for Emily's dolls. She was having too much fun playing to stop and visit the bathroom, and had an accident in the homemade doll's crib.

One moment I was laughing and playing with her, the next moment I was yelling at her. Telling her that she knew better. Telling her that she was too big to have these accidents anymore. She ran crying into the bathroom as I followed her in. While I rinsed the clothes and crib in the sink, Emily sat on the toilet sobbing, "I'm sorry, Mom. I'm sorry, Mom," over and over.

What's clear to me even now is the lucidity with which I observed all this. Thoughts came into my head; I simply observed them. Emily cried; I simply observed it. I gave her a stern lecture; I simply observed the words coming out of my mouth. I was doing what I had been practicing: the art of self-observation. I was detached from the events in an uncaring and unloving way.

This is not what I was striving for in my personal practice.

I've found that the art of observation, of expanding awareness, needs a tether. It needs to be rooted in some behavior that allows for a connection to the world. Otherwise, the practice of self-observation runs the risk of being clinical, cold, and impersonal. Or it runs the risk of being some neat little escape from the irritations of life. And this can cause others pain, as it did my daughter.

The tether for self-observation can be secured in the next step of the **EASE** process: Self-reflection.

Experience answers the question "What are my thoughts, feelings and actions?"

Awareness answers the question, "What else is there?"

Self-reflection answers the question "How do I want to be in this world?"

At this stage, the **EASE** process makes a significant shift: a shift from cognitive, intellectual exploration to the realm of the heart; a shift from passive observation and expansion to active creation; a shift from random chance to purposeful alignment.

The other night I went into the bathroom to brush my teeth before bed. Emily had just done the same a short while ago. Looking into the mirror I couldn't help but notice that Emily had probably enjoyed playing a game while brushing her teeth. The mirror was covered with toothpaste specks. I could barely make out my reflection because of the distortion. I was ready for bed and wasn't interested in cleaning at this point, so I just adjusted my eyes to consciously look at the reflection behind the toothpaste dots. The specks were easier to focus on, since it covered a larger area, but I found I could make out my true reflection if I just looked closely enough.

Self-reflection is the process of looking into your heart, seeing what values move you, and then incorporating those more fully into your life. Self-reflection is a way of choosing your own passion or vision statement. It's consciously refining a given characteristic. That value, trait or characteristic may not be prevalent now, but through focused attention it can be consciously cultivated.

The formulation for this step came from an interesting discussion I had with the then-President of Dupont Pharmaceuticals, Nick Teti.

I was at the Marriott Hotel, attached to the Philadelphia International Airport, attending another meeting with Dupont's Integrated Healthcare team. I was still new to Dupont, having worked there less than two years. After the meeting finished, I walked across the lobby, rolling my suitcase, heading towards the terminal for my flight. I crossed paths with Nick, who had also attended the meeting.

After the traditional small talk, Nick asked me a question that would have been a great setup had I been willing to take the bait. "Megan," he asked, "what would you like to do in this organization?" At another time I may have jumped for joy and gave a great rendition of my career aspirations and why I was suited for such grand endeavors. Now, I found myself cringing inside because he had unwittingly hit a sore spot. I had no idea what I wanted to do, where I was going, or even if I was in the right organization. In fact, I was completely lost.

Not knowing how to answer, I asked him a different question. I asked, "Did you always know you wanted to be president?" His answer kept my mind and heart busy all the way back to Massachusetts, and then some. His reply, "It isn't what you want to *do* that is important, it is how you want to *be*."

A light bulb went off in my head.

From childhood, we're asked, "What do you want to do when you grow up?" I found the question irritating, perhaps because I never had a clear answer.

There are a unique few who have always known their chosen profession. For the rest of us, life's twists and turns, everyday decisions and minor coincidences have brought us to our current spot.

The question "What do you want to do?" sets up a future-oriented focus, a striving that says implicitly, at least, that all isn't right where you are. That some pinnacle needs to be reached before you can say, "I'm where I'm meant to be."

Nick's answer—focusing on behavior and values instead of a nonstop career ladder—had a profound impact on me, shifting internal gears.

This is much simpler than trying to orchestrate the direction of your life's work. Setting up internal values that drive daily behavior can be done here and now—no need to wait for some ethereal moment in the future.

In a prelude to *The Dance*, Oriah Mountain Dreamer posed the following question: "What if it truly doesn't matter what you do but how you do whatever you do?"

Great question. How do you do whatever you do?

This way of looking at your work creates a personal vision of how you want to be in relation to work. The term "vision statement" is well known in the corporate world. Sometimes it can have a bad connotation. For some organizations, a vision statement is nothing more than the executives coming back from a retreat and making a grand statement to the organization that sounds suspiciously like all other vision statements. Or, the employees are asked to partake in a visioning statement, which ring hollow when words and actions are not in concert with the supposed vision.

For the S step in the **EASE** process, you commit to a personal statement deciding how you want to be in this world. This can be called your passion statement or passion words, rather than your vision statement, since the term "vision" refers to some distance thing being viewed from a present vantage point. Rather, a passion statement is a strong, emotional commitment to a way of being. The passion keeps you committed to the concept even when it is easier to walk away or be something other than what you committed to.

The S step of the Ease process correlates to one of Yoga's eight principal limbs, the principal of moral restraint *(yama)* and observances *(niyamas)*. Patanjali's moral restraints include non-harming *(ahimsa)*, truthfulness *(satya)*, non-stealing *(asteya)*, chastity *(brahmacarya)*, and greedlessness *(aparigraha)*. The moral observances include purity *(saucha)*, contentment *(santosa)*, purification *(tapas)*, self-study *(svadhyaya)* and surrender to the divine *(Isvara pranidhana)*.

Rather than subscribing to a certain moral code, the S step asks you to look inside yourself and find those values that resonate with you. Ultimately, all values lead in one of two directions. Values either lead to more openness, acceptance and love, or they lead to confinement, close-mindedness and fear.

Mahatma Gandhi is one of the most powerful examples in recent history for strength of intentional behavior. He was committed to a cause: liberating India from English rule. He was even more committed to the behavior that would lead his people to freedom: nonviolence. No matter what horrible conditions Gandhi was subjected to, nonviolence was his personal stake in the ground. This was a quality, a way of being, a personal passion so strong it was immovable. In the face of violence, fear and aggression, Gandhi chose nonviolence time and time again. It was Gandhi's personal statement of who he was, and from the position of strength and fortitude he moved mountains.

How do you choose your own passion statement? You choose by noticing what qualities inspire or resonate with you. Remember, self-reflection answers the question "How do I want to be in this world?" Answers could be:

> *Loving*
>
> *Courageous*
>
> *Forgiving*
>
> *Brave*
>
> *Accepting*
>
> *Purposeful*
>
> *Kind*
>
> *Open*
>
> *Adventurous*
>
> *Willing*
>
> *Playful*

A passion statement would simply be the words you are trying to bring to life. For example, on the airplane after having the discussion with Nick, I chose the following passion statement: Live, love and learn.

You're not aiming for poetry or rocket science. It's not the words that count; it's the feeling and depth that is behind them.

The purpose of the **S** step in the **EASE** process is to be able to see how you currently define yourself, and then clarify how you would choose to be. The self-reflection stage, the **S** step, is crucial. It's a definition of how you want to be.

Frame Your World

I was getting ready for work one morning, so I glanced at the clock to see if I was on schedule. My husband's clock said 6:56 A.M., leaving me feeling hurried to get out the door by 7:00. I doubled checked the time with the clock on my side of the bed. It read 6:53. Phew, I had plenty of time.

I really doubt that three minutes made much of a difference at all. What happened in my brain is that I looked at 6:56 and rounded it up to 7:00. Translation—I'd better get moving. My clock, at 6:53, was closer in the rounding process to 6:50, ten minutes until departing time. Translation—I have plenty of time. What's interesting was the effect these three minutes of time, more or less, had on my mental state. Three minutes less, I felt hurried. Three minutes more and I felt relaxed and unrushed.

But isn't the concept of time an absolute? What time was correct? Which reaction was correct?

In the beginning of the **EASE** process, I discussed the fact that your experience is framed. We're hard-wired over time to construct a framework with which to decipher and make sense of the world. This framing naturally limits and confines what and how we see and becomes an expression of who we think we are. The way in which I viewed time is an example of creating this kind of limitation.

In yogic terms, deeply ingrained personality traits are called *samskaras.*

The classic example used to describe *samskara* is the action of waves upon water. When water is still, the view to the bottom is clear (when your mind is clear you can see the true nature of your Self). When waves churn up the water (or when thoughts churn in the mind) it makes it difficult to see clearly. Over time, the waves make a seemingly more permanent structure in the sand—ripples and sculptures made by the action above. In the mind, similar patterns of behavior are borne out of experience, thoughts, and actions. These patterns seem integral to who we are—a part of our character. Feeling rushed by the clock is an example of such a character trait many of us feel in this busy world.

We are not the patterns, however. Just like the sand, molded by waves, can be remolded through a new wave action, so too can you re-form your view of the world—even with a concept as seemingly concrete as time.

The act of self-reflection in the S step of the **EASE** process, and of choosing a passion statement, is framing your world. It's setting up a construct with which to view the world. However, instead of the unconscious framing most of us meander through life with, this is a conscious, deliberate framing.

In her book, *A Simpler Way,* Margaret Wheatley talks about life as a cooperative endeavor, rather than competitive in nature. Wheatley challenges the commonly held view of the Darwinian concept—that the strong survive; the weak eventually fade away through evolutionary selection. Her suggestion is to look at the world as a cooperative endeavor, that the act of belonging to a world community means that we are all interdependent, and therefore cooperation is the model of universal evolution.

It's unlikely that a bird considers whether her actions are cooperative or competitive. She just does her thing. What's fascinating is that when a human labels something as a "competition," it sets up a whole set of attitudes that foster certain actions. When a human calls something "cooperation" it sets up a completely different response. It's the mind that makes the decision, and in that decision the reality is created.

That's why it's so important to deliberately choose the frame though which you view the world.

In *Walden*, Thoreau wrote, "The mass of men lead lives of quiet desperation." Through years and years of unconscious conditioning, we shaped our world—and our relationship to it—into an automatic response. We've become slaves to accepted norms, and that quiet desperation is a reminder to wake up.

Now is a good time to switch from autopilot to being awake with your responses. If you haven't done so already, choose one, two, or three words that frame the way you wish to be in the world.

Join the Inner Peace Corps

September 11th, 2001. In an instant, our sense of security became forever contaminated.

Besides the sickening sight of a plane smashing into the World Trade Center, one picture stands out in my mind. Watching the news coverage soon after the event, I saw paper floating through the air along with smoke and debris, like streaming confetti in some horrid parade.

Watching the paper drift down, it dawned on me that five minutes earlier these papers were deemed important, perhaps highly confidential and significant to the business at hand. They meant something to someone. They had a purpose.

No longer. The paper was transformed into trash as our priorities—and the world's—refocused on what really mattered: Family. Love. Hope. Support. Compassion. Life itself.

I was out at the library with my children when I heard the news that the World Trade Center had been hit. At first I thought a small plane pilot had lost control of the airplane. Walking across the street to get a smoothie for the kids and a tea for myself at the local coffee shop, I saw the pictures on the television and knew the second plane had hit as well. This was no accident.

Like people around the country, I gathered with others for support that night. A group of us came together for a meditation held close to my hometown in central Massachusetts. The mere act of coming together held some semblance of forward action, countering the feeling of great sadness. In an impromptu ceremony, we lit candles and said prayers for those most closely impacted by the event, for loved ones who were traveling, and for our leaders who were responsible for deciding actions yet to come.

Later that week Gen Kelsang Chöma, an American Buddhist nun, spoke at the same spot about hope. She said this tragic event could be transformed by galvanizing an inner resolve to end suffering. Chöma suggested that we each make a pledge to join the "Inner Peace Corps."

Chöma taught that September 11th could catalyze a commitment to living inner priorities every day. Tragic events have a way of turning you on your head, searing your mind with the reminder that life is unpredictable and precious. These moments slap us with the realization that life is not to be taken for granted.

Consider the following pledge in response to Chöma's offer to join the Inner Peace Corps:

- For each person you pass, resolve to smile peace.

- For each display of anger, including your own, resolve to let go and hear the heart's whisper of another way.

- For tears of grief, resolve to embrace compassion.

- For deep fear in search of safety, resolve to strengthen an inner connection.

∞ For searing pain in search of retribution, resolve to mirror understanding.

∞ For each comment that foretells of future doom and gloom, resolve to speak of hope, of light, of possibilities.

∞ Let each passing plane be a reminder of this inner commitment.

Use the memory of September 11th to mold your mind in a positive way. When a plane passes overhead, breathe in your passion words. The **S** step in the **EASE** is remembering what you value. What is that for you?

∞

Triangulation

A country restaurant served an unexpected French cuisine. Although the food was a beauty, the cook was a beast. He had the stereotypical disposition of a temperamental chef. His cooking was superb, but his tableside manner was brisk, bordering on rude. If you wore perfume or washed your clothes with a scented detergent, or were deemed "rude" by some unknown rules, you were asked to leave. He was a fantastic French chef, but you didn't mess with him.

These are the types of people that test our mindset, every day and in every way. The ground-shaking events like September 11th do not come every day, thank God. The work that strengthens our minds in preparation for such a devastating day happens in the commonplace interactions of asking the moody cook to toast our bagel.

What shapes our mind most significantly are the repetitive, and seemingly insignificant, daily events. How we manage these sets the tone for how we respond to global, earth-shattering events.

The little things are like a dress rehearsal for our mind for opening night.

This is the idea of triangulation. Global Positioning Satellites (GPS) use this concept to find out where you are and the best way to go to get somewhere else. It's based on simple geometry. If you know two points you can solve for the third point.

Real life gives us the opportunity to know ourselves through the triangulation of relationships.

If I say I'm going to be loving, yet bark out orders at work and get mad at the temperamental cook, then these are the two points that can be used to modify the third: my mind.

In terms of the **EASE** process, the S for self-reflection shows you that your mind is much more malleable than you may have thought. The point of triangulation is to use everyday circumstances to gauge where your mind is now. During the course of your day, notice when you're living your passion statement and when you're not. In this way, you become better acquainted with the workings of your mind, body and emotions, so that you will be able to modify them more effectively.

If you know where you are, and know where you want to go, then your relationships and daily irritations can be the true terrain for testing.

If you explore love only in the safety of an ideal, it's like reading a map without ever walking over the earth.

It's worthwhile examining a topographical map before planning a hiking trip. Just don't confuse the map of the path with the path itself. Managing the up and down terrain of the real world is always more challenging. In other words, it's always more difficult to live love than it is to speak of it as an ideal.

The Heart's Center

Scrubbing the toilet is not my favorite activity. I doubt it's on anybody's top-ten list of enjoyable tasks. But in the family scheme of things, it seems that I invariably end up with the job, and I resent it.

One memorable weekend I was spending a Saturday cleaning the house. Chores, errands and scrubbing the toilet end up being weekend activities. So much for recreation.

I was fuming, feeling that I was shouldering the lion's share of household chores. This resentment gives great energy to do housework, but it's not very constructive. I huffed and puffed through the house, finally making it to the bathroom. I decided to try my passion statement on for size. How could I bring to life the words live, love and learn while scrubbing the toilet?

I worked hard at controlling the resentment. I would try to think "loving" thoughts, but then the angry thoughts would come to refuel the embers. One thought pattern in particular would send me down the path of resentment—that my husband said he just couldn't remember to scrub the toilet.

The toilet can get downright disgusting. My husband claims that no matter how bad it gets, he simply does not notice and it does not occur to him to scrub the bowl. Well, I tested that theory, and no matter how bad I let it get, he did not scrub it.

This thought kept my resentment going that day: if you relieve yourself standing up, how on earth can you not see that the bowl needs cleaning? Bottom line, I wasn't buying his story. He was sticking to it though, and we had come to an impasse. I complained; he listed all the other household chores he had done.

I gave up on the matter, as you eventually do after a certain number of years in marriage. I resigned myself to the fact that toilet scrubbing was my chore and I ungraciously took it on.

One day that all changed. I was in my home office, doing work on my computer. The house was empty. What a gift silence can be. I enjoyed being able to focus entirely on the work at hand. I only left the office for two reasons: to get another sweater and put on some hot tea. The house seemed chilly and my cold fingers had a hard time moving over the keyboard.

At the end of the day, my family returned and I was pleased with my progress at work. When my husband stepped in from outside, he noticed the house was cold. A good deal of our heat comes from the wood stove in the basement. Since the thermostat is set low, it gets quite chilly before the heat kicks on. Joe asked me if I put wood in the stove, which of course I hadn't. "How could you forget to put wood on the fire when you felt how cold the house was?" he accused me. "Don't ever complain to me about forgetting to scrub the toilet again."

Touché, Joe.

It honestly did not cross my mind to put wood into the stove, even though I was cold. It dawned on me that it honestly didn't cross Joe's mind to scrub the toilet either. I believed his story now, since I had a context with which to understand it.

I'm still the family toilet scrubber these days—I'm trying to teach my three-year-old how to hold the brush—but I'm not resentful about it now.

A funny thing about passion statements—they take on a whole new meaning when you actually experience the words rather than holding on to an intellectual interpretation of their meaning.

Once I understood my husband's perspective through my own experience of the wood stove, there was an inner click that was experiential, not theoretical. And then it was easier to stick to my passion statement of "love."

The idea of living a passion statement has an inner quality associated with it that is independent of the intellectual understanding of the word.

In their book, *The Heartmath Solution*, Doc Childre and Howard Martin talk about the associated feelings in the heart that accompany emotional states. They use biofeedback to show how heart rate and other physiologic factors change when we engage the heart. Just thinking of your pet or strolling along a warm beach changes your mindset.

There is an intelligence in the heart and body that is different than the thinking mind that we are so familiar with. In this society we are less comfortable with the terrain of the heart. Whether it's scrubbing toilets or hugging a baby, enlisting your heart to participate will help you become more familiar with changing your mindset.

Review your passion statement again. Look at the words closely; breathe them into your body. What do they mean to you? How do they feel in your body?

When you're having difficulty living them, just notice. You will have a "eureka" moment when an opportunity comes along to show you what that passion statement means in relation to the action you should take.

Having the head and the heart work towards a common goal is incredibly powerful. In the S step of the **EASE** process, self-reflection on the heart is particularly called for. As you begin to consider different passion words that resonate for you, you can notice the different associated feelings they have in your body and in your heart.

What is the difference for example, between contentment and ecstasy? Between love and caring? Between trust and acceptance? Between compassion and empathy? Between patience and passivity?

Each of these words has an intellectual connotation for us, as well as an emotional feeling associated with it. You can use the discriminating mind to tease out the differences or you can just notice for yourself how you feel, down to every detail, how these emotions live in your body.

Open to Change and Growth

When I first became a Yoga teacher, I wondered how I would fit in. My perception about how a teacher should be did not fit how I was. Rather than quiet and pensive, I was often boisterous and loud with a deep hearty laugh that didn't quite fit my framework of a serene and still yogi.

When you begin living your passion statement, trying to be a certain quality, you will eventually run up against your preconceived idea of what that trait should look like.

Let's pretend that you decided you wanted to be more patient. What does it mean to be patient when your 16-year-old son just came home drunk? How does patience work when you are grabbing the hand of your toddler before she burns her hand on the stove?

Invariably, when you choose a passion statement, you're working within your own preconceived definition. Like my view of the perfect Yoga teacher, your passion statement will need to expand in context to the environment you are in. Patience doesn't mean being a wimp. Being a Yoga teacher doesn't mean you always have to talk in a quiet, meditative voice. The passion words you chose are big enough to hold every circumstance.

∞

Die

Let's play a game. Pretend that you're old, very old. You've lived a long and wonderful life, and you know that tonight you'll die. You have no unresolved fear or dread about your death; you're ready. You spend this time quietly contemplating your life. As you review your life certain words come to mind to describe the quality of the life you have lead. What words would you like to come to mind? What way of being fills your heart with contentment?

The issue is not what you *did* with your life, but how you *were* in your life. How would you be in this world now if you had this quality?

What this comes down to is how you define success.

The idea of defining success came from a seminar I attended at my favorite bookstore. This is one of those all-too-rare bookstores that is still family-owned. It has an eclectic style with a wonderful restaurant where one can nurse a cup of coffee for hours while thumbing through books. I could spend all day here.

A motivational speaker was on the agenda that morning. Sipping my coffee, I listened to his ideas about how to be successful, how to bring into your life all that you desire, how to make things happen. Being in sales, I was very used to this type of presentation. A question came from the audience, "How would you define success?"

This is a great question that we can all ask ourselves. What does success look like for you? Most tend to approach the question from the think-and-grow-rich mindset. That is, if we had a certain job, salary, or spouse we would be successful. If we lived in the right house, in the right neighborhood, with the right car in the three-car garage then we have reached success.

There is a much simpler way to gauge success: the contentment quotient.

We have all known people who have amassed a lot of stuff. They have all the latest that money can buy. However, they still don't seem very content. At times they are happy, as we all are, but this underlying contentment quotient is missing. How content do you feel with your life no matter what the external circumstances?

Take ten minutes and write a paragraph from the perspective of the end of your life, a life you deemed successful. A life you were contented with. After you finish writing, a short paragraph or a long story, read through it. Read it with your heart, not with your intellect. What theme comes through? Are there words that are repeated throughout, a quality?

The self-reflection step in the **EASE** process begins a conscious, deliberate way of life that you would choose to create for yourself and others. It's putting a stake in the ground saying HERE! HERE is where I choose to be. This is what I call success. This quality, this way of being is the core to center my life around.

This concept could be viewed as Pollyanna-ish. It could be viewed as a nice way to live, but not terribly applicable to the "real" world. Let me show you how I used this concept.

Do you remember when I told you that I had to work on a project with a man who saw everything differently than me? We would invariably take opposing sides on just about any topic that arose. During the course of self-observation and working through the **EASE** process, I realized that I could not hear a word he was saying. Quite literally, I could not process the words he was speaking. The frustration and anger blocked out any semblance of two-way communication.

My personal passion words are "live, love and learn." Three simple words that mean much more than the thirteen letters that comprise them. It was clear that my interactions with this man were in no way congruent with my personal vision of how I wanted to live my life. Love is certainly large enough to hold a disagreement, but love was not what I was feeling when working with him.

At night, when I had physical and emotional distance from the situation, I began to cultivate my desired intentions. I relaxed my body, conjured the feeling of love, and then applied it to a mental picture of the man I disagreed with. In the next meeting, I could hear what he said. I still disagreed with his opinions, and his general philosophy, but I was connected. I could hear. I could smile. I could live the way I had chosen.

Here are the specific steps for you to be able to do the same thing: First, breathe into your entire body, bringing awareness to your entire being. Relaxing into this, notice your breathing, watching it coming in and out of your body. Settle into an even rhythm. Then, bring your passion word into your body with the breath. If, for example, you have chosen "love" as the quality you wish to bring to life, breathe love into your entire body. Picture it as a warm yellow light. Or picture it as a feeling when holding someone dear. Or hear it as a melody that vibrates through your body. What does love look like to you? Touch that and spread it through your being. When you feel connected, gently bring to mind the person you would like to bring this quality to. Remember, you're not changing another into something you would prefer. You are opening yourself to be the way you choose to be.

If this is really difficult because you have a deep-seated frustration with this individual or situation, begin first by using a situation where you truly feel love for another. For example, perhaps you have a personal mentor in business that your love naturally extends to. Practice here first if that works for you.

Summary

- Self-reflection answers the question "How do you want to be in this world?" It's a conscious framing of your world instead of accepting an automated reaction to external events.

- Self-reflection is heart-centered; it's not an intellectual exercise. Take time to hear the heart's whisper through the roar of everyday life.

- The frames you use to see the world are mutable. You do have the ability to shape how you want to be. There is freedom in this understanding and application; you're not a prisoner within yourself.

- Use your everyday life to see yourself clearly, especially with the people you find most aggravating.

- Take time to define what success means to you.

- Your ability to live your passion words will grow as you expand your understanding of them past a preconceived definition.

Step Four

Elect

Liquid Gold

My sister used to work in day care, so she had plenty of experience with children before having her own. Watching other people's children wasn't the same as being a parent, we decided one day while commiserating about the difficulties of childrearing. "I was the greatest mother before I had children," she said.

It's always easier to *say* what you will do, rather than do what you say.

The second **E** in **EASE**, **E2**, stands for elect. The last step of the **EASE** process is to elect or choose in a given moment to act in accordance with your passion statement. Passion words may be simple to say, but they're not always easy to do. Just as my sister and I had grand ideas on how to be the best mother, it remained only a theory until we had children of our own. Only then could we use the experience as a testing ground for our beliefs.

Before I had children of my own, for example, I swore that I would never use the television as a baby-sitter. I envisioned a stimulating, constructive environment where I provided all sorts of educational opportunities for my offspring. Now, dying for a moment of peace and quiet to do something exciting like fold laundry, I'm happily throwing in the latest Disney flick. Enjoy, kids. Don't bother Mommy. . . .

When you set out your passion statement in S, although it may resonate soundly with your heart, it's only a theory until you encounter the circumstance that allows you to express it. **E2** is taking a belief, a heart's desire, and recreating it on a moment-by-moment basis. The way to know love is to discover it in every moment, not just when a circumstance is "loving." The application and deeper definition of love comes when the circumstances are anything but loving, yet you choose it anyway.

My husband, Joe, makes maple syrup. In fact, as I write this he's heading off to collect the sap from the trees, and I'll run down to the sugarhouse every fifteen minutes or so to check on the boiling process. Cold nights and warm days in early spring create a flow of sap up the trunk from the roots of the tree.

The sap looks just like water. When you drink it, you can taste a hint of sweetness, which is why it's called sweet water. It makes a great cup of tea. The only step needed to transform sap into syrup is to boil off the water. Constantly. Continually. Mother Nature provides everything that's needed for the final product from the beginning. The boiling condenses the sap until it yields pure maple syrup. Liquid gold.

It takes forty gallons of sap to make one gallon of syrup, so the process isn't quick. Joe started boiling at 10:00 this morning, and it's now almost 8:00 at night. He'll probably be at it until midnight or so.

The sap-to-syrup process is like the **E2** step. **E2** is the process of taking your passion words from imagination to creation in day-to-day life. It's not some magical overnight transformation.

Just like the sap has to boil continually, your intentions have to be tended in order to cultivate that which you would like to see in your life. Just like planting a seed doesn't yield a flower overnight, your intentions need attention.

There are times when you'll get frustrated, thinking that you should be making more "progress" in relation to some expected outcome. Remember, though, just like the sap has everything right from the beginning to make maple syrup, you already have what you're trying so hard to get. It's all there already.

It's a New Year Every Day

At a recent conference, best-selling author Seth Godin shared an interesting fact. He said that if you weren't in the habit of reading a newspaper by the time you turned 30, chances are you would never acquire the habit. The death spiral of the newspaper industry is attributed to this fact; the younger generation hasn't developed the ritual of daily newspaper reading. We can see this truth in our own experience. Many times ingrained patterns become fixed in our lives very early on. Breaking these habits or starting a new one takes effort, as anyone who has made a New Year's resolution can attest to.

The first step **E** in the **EASE** process, looking closely at your experience, sets the stage for recognizing habits. The **A** step, expanding your awareness, helps expand your view to include new options outside your current experience. During the **S** step of self-reflection, the focus changes from automatic reactions to determining a conscious response. In **E2** you practice bringing these conscious values to life every day, which establishes positive habits.

The energy brought about by a New Year's resolution is false. We fool ourselves into thinking that the New Year is a clean slate; time to start anew. The idea that New Year's Day has some special magic for turning over a new leaf is based on a cultural belief that January 1 is a new beginning.

In Yoga philosophy, time is simply the sequence of each moment, which is forever new. This now that you're in is new. So is this now. And this. And this. On and on, each moment is a New Year. What we fail to recognize is that every day, every moment, is a New Year. It's never too late to start reading the paper, or to live your values.

You'll find that when you try to implement your passion words in E2, circumstance plays a huge role in your ability to act the way you've deemed important. With some people, for example, you'll have an easy time being patient. With others, just the way they talk will grate on your nerves, making you impatient and short-tempered. It's just like being on a diet. Sometimes it's easy to eat well, but your resolve is tested when your favorite chocolate cake is plunked in front of you. Like a New Year's resolution, it's important to keep reinforcing your commitment in E2.

Some people tend to berate themselves when they can't stick to a New Year's resolution or to E2, as if their willpower is somehow lacking and that it has nothing at all to do with circumstances. Others tend to do the opposite, placing the blame on circumstances rather than on willpower. The ability to consistently live espoused values is a combination of commitment, circumstance and cultivation.

You're not an island. You're part of a complex system of interrelated influences. Therefore, making a decision to be a certain way is strongly affected by the context in which you find yourself. The impact of a system is most strongly felt in the beginning part of the self-leadership process. After all, the goal of the **EASE** process is to break out of automatic responses to the external environment and create a self-directed way of living that honors you and recognizes the reality of the situation you're in.

A given outcome is not affected solely by your actions. It's a combined result of everybody who's even remotely connected to the situation. Your environment and your response to that environment co-create the moment you're in now, and the future that is yet to come.

This interconnectedness is evident in something as simple as drinking a glass of water. Bringing a glass to your lips, think about the history of the water within. At one time molecules from this same water were in the sky as moisture, perhaps from a time long ago. They came together in a cloud and rained down to earth. Seeping through the soil, the water was absorbed by the roots of a tree. The water went through the tree and was used to produce fruit, and eaten by a person. The water traveled through the body, and came out as sweat through the skin. Returning to the atmosphere, the cycle starts all over again. When you drink a glass of water, you do more than simply rehydrate. The history of every molecule of water becomes part of you.

So, just do the best you can, and know that the outcome of your **E2** step won't look exactly as you planned. Be patient. Keep at it. Eventually you'll have more control over the circumstances than they have over you.

The Nature of the Mind

While searching to understand my own thoughts, I've noticed a pattern that helps implement E2. This framework is not part of a specific philosophical body; it's just my own observations of self. See how it works for you.

I've segmented the mind into four categories. For ease of understanding, compare it to the parts of a computer. The four categories are: foreground, background, memory and CPU.

There are times when your thoughts are focused and busy on the day-to-day activities of life. This is like the foreground of the computer. It's like actively working on a Microsoft® Excel spreadsheet or a document in Microsoft® Word. Taking a shower, writing a list of things to do and paying the bills are examples of your mind working on the foreground. Right now I'm working in the foreground of my mind as I write these words.

Below the level of the foreground is the background. I can be working with the computer in Word, when a bell signals that the mail has been received in the background. I can also be doing a task in the foreground, but my mind has a certain amount of attention going towards something else in the background, such as what I should cook for dinner.

Many techniques in mediation and Yoga are designed to focus the mind completely, so there is no split between the foreground and background. It's in this space of concentrated attention that the power of the mind is expanded. When it comes to the E2 step, the background space can be used as a behind-the-scenes assistant to living your day-to-day passion words.

For example, I've been lightly holding onto a general idea of what the next step of this book is going to look like. I've allowed the concept for this chapter to stay in the background. While I'm going through my everyday activities in the foreground of my mind, an activity will set off a bell in my brain, saying "Oh, this connects nicely with the next chapter in the book." When I actually put the idea into writing on my word processor, it's moved from the background into the foreground.

There are times when your passion words are in the foreground of your mind; there are times when they are in the background. As long as they are somewhere, it's a good thing. Sometimes it works well to have the passion words in the forefront of your mind, acting them out in a given moment. There are times when holding them in the foreground feels much too forced and strained. Then it's better to hold onto the concept lightly in the background and let it percolate. The trick is not to let your passion words percolate too long without action, or the energy to instill them into reality just boils off.

We can only hold so much stuff in the background. Just like the computer can only have so many programs open, I've found I can only work on holding so many things in the back of my head. If I don't lightly hold the writing questions in my head, the writing won't come to the foreground to get actually written. The same is true of your passion words. If you don't keep them at or close to the top of your mind, they will fade.

Below the foreground is the background. Below the background is memory. The computer has files stored away that you have probably forgotten about. In your memory there are patterns and ways of being that are hidden from you directly. It's the realm where you're not acting consciously for a particular reason; you have something ingrained in your behavior that goes way back. Too much stored in a computer's memory affects the functioning of everyday work, slowing it down. The old files need to be archived for optimal performance. Your mind can have old baggage from long ago that's affecting the energy you have available for today. Many times before you can effectively bring E2 into action, past memories need to be properly sorted and archived.

The deepest part of the mind is what I call silence. It's the most difficult to put into words or to ascribe attributes to. I compare it to the CPU of the computer because this silence really is the source of power within each of us. It's a still point that's before any thought or action, but it accompanies everything. Within the loudest cacophony is the sound of this silence.

Here's an example of it in action. I was driving home the other night and my car—which I affectionately call Chitty Chitty Bang Bang—decided to get temperamental. The headlights kept going on and off. One minute I was driving down the deserted country road with the headlights on, the next I was in complete darkness as the lights went out. I wasn't sure what to do. My mind in the foreground was busy formulating what to do. I was searching my background and memory for suggestions on what could cause this. Then out of nowhere—out of silence—came a thought: turn off the heat. I did and the problem went away. Who would have guessed?

You can use this interpretation of the mind to guide your own exploration of your thoughts. Patanjali gave a different description of the thought-waves *(chitta)* in the mind *(vritti)*. He said that there are five kinds of thoughts: right knowledge, wrong knowledge, verbal delusion, sleep and memory. The thoughts that move us deeper into ignorance, or away from our true Self are painful, and those that move us closer to our true nature are not painful.

Whether you examine your thoughts using the computer analogy or using Patanjali's classification of thoughts doesn't matter. Regardless of the method, looking closely at your thoughts allow you to see their nature. You need not be a slave to thoughts once you see them clearly. In fact, thoughts are a strong way to influence E2. As you think, so you act. Changing thoughts change the behavior.

When you begin trying to re-form your mind and your actions in E2, I'd be surprised if you hit a bull's eye right away, acting every moment in concert with your passion words. In actuality, the process is more like successive approximation.

Successive approximation is the process of moving towards a desired state one step at a time. You keep guessing at what you think the right action is, noticing the results you get, and then try again, coming closer and closer to the goal. As you move through successive approximation, you begin to see different layers of your mind.

I watched Picabo Street fly down the mountain during the Winter Olympics. The physical stamina and dedication of the Olympic athletes is always an inspiration to me. I noticed a blue line on the snow that was weaving snakelike through the course. The commentator said these lines helped the skier see the course in shady areas. It kept them on track.

Successive approximation of the **E2** step is like the skiers trying to hit the line on the slope: when you're on it you know. When you are living your values, you know it from the inside.

According to Native American myth, pure maple syrup used to flow out of the trees without any work. Then a trickster in the tribe, Glooskap, poured river water into the top of the trees, making the syrup run thin. After that, the sap had to be boiled down and concentrated before enjoying the syrup. Glooskap said his clan would be better able to appreciate the sweetness of the syrup when contrasted with the watery sap.

Sometimes I think stress and anxiety exist so one can better appreciate the stillness of the inner line.

∞

Cleaning Out the Closets

The beginning of spring in New England is always a touch-and-go war between the seasons. Today it was over fifty degrees and sunny; tomorrow snow is predicted. The ice in the ground melts with the warm sun, creating mud piles my three-year-old loves to stomp through, and then leave dirt trails through the house. The next day the messy mud may be frozen solid into difficult peaks and grooves.

Spring is a messy, in-between time. My children's closets are way too full as I try to find room for ski suits while digging through packed-away clothes to find lighter garb for the warm weather. My daughter was outside in a tee shirt today; tomorrow she might need her ski jacket. It makes for a congested house.

Transition times are awkward. Old stuff is still there; new stuff is moving in. Both demand attention. In the E2 step, when you make the shift from automatic responses to making conscious choices about how you want to be, it can be awkward. Old, familiar patterns are overlaid with new, unknown roles.

Here are a few tips for approaching this in-between season:

Accept the mess. Life won't be as neat and predictable as it was before; it'll be messy. Since you are trying to change ingrained patterns of behavior, frustration and stress will inevitably crop up. Temper it with the knowledge that the mess is a natural part of the process.

Trust the process. Despite the mess, know that patterns and new order will prevail. Just like sap turns to maple syrup, your conscious actions will eventually have an impact. It won't stay messy forever.

Let it go. You're not superhuman. When you take on a new way of being, you simply cannot do it all at once. Just do the best you can.

Take it on. It's sometimes easier to stick with the known rather than enter new territory. Grab onto the new challenge of changing your intentions with at least curiosity if not enthusiasm.

The *Tao Teh Ching*, a classic book of poetry and a guide to spiritual development over 2,000 years old, states, "To realize that our knowledge is ignorance, this is a noble insight."

And there's nothing like a grand transition to remind us of our own ignorance. But when the closets are all cleaned, and the transition is complete, you'll have found new treasures to take with you for the next seasonal cycle sure to come.

Roadblocks to Success

I've been told that to be a true coach, I need to complete a certain education. I've been told that to teach Yoga properly, I must have a specific school certification. I've been told that to participate in a leadership conference, I need to have the title of executive director. I've been told that in order to be a professional speaker, I must be a member in a national association.

Life is difficult enough without people telling you what you *have* to do to be worthy of something. Sometimes the loudest voice saying that you're not worthy is your own.

When you find that you are unable to live the values in the E2 step that you would like to have in your life, anger, impatience and self-flagellation can arise. These feelings can be harmful since they're so potent and can eat away at inner peace. But the energy of anger and impatience can be transformed into a strong catalyst for creating inner resolve. They can be used to find your own voice.

When you are having difficulty living your values, mentors and role models can be a wonderful antidote for the anger and impatience that may arise. Who is being the way you would like to be?

Anthony Hopkins and Alec Baldwin starred in a movie called *The Edge*. Hopkins, a quiet genius who also happens to be a billionaire, is lost in the Alaskan wilderness with Baldwin, a hip fashion photographer. After their plane crashes, they strike out to find safety. Along the way, a man-killer bear finds and follows them, hoping to eat them for lunch.

Hopkins rallies Baldwin's enthusiasm to fight the beast, rather than to simply give up. He tells a story about how someone had killed a bear with a simple spear made out of wood. Hopkins coaches Baldwin to repeat the phrase "What one man can do, another can do," ramping up volume and enthusiasm until both were yelling their support of this impossible task.

You guessed it; they killed the bear with a simple spear made out of a stick.

OK, so that's a tad Hollywood. But having someone as a role model simply means that you see what they've accomplished and from that, you can see possibilities for yourself.

In Yoga, there exists a triangle of forces—called *gunas*—that can either help or hinder your progress towards a specific goal. Whether that goal is to be a rich businessperson, fight a man-eating bear, or become a liberated soul, these qualities move together day in and day out.

The forces that compose the universe—and our mind—are: *sattwa*, *rajas*, and *tamas*. Here's an example of how they play together. While taking a shower you have an inspiration about a new project. Thinking about it fills your mind with excitement. This is the quality of *sattwa*, the essence of a form or the inspiration behind it. It's the creative juice before the work begins.

After being inspired, you decide to do some research on the Internet. The idea you came up with has some serious flaws. It will take a lot of hard work to make the idea come to life. The earlier excitement you felt is turning into heaviness as you see all the work that needs to be done. "Why bother?" you question as the excitement wanes. This is the energy of *tamas*, the obstacle that has to be overcome to realize the inspiration. *Tamas* feels heavy in your body, like the energy of inertia.

You decide to undertake the project anyway, even though it means a lot of hard work. You work late, your family helps out, and your friends join in. There is an energy of commitment, of dedication to the original inspiration that overtakes the inertia. This is the energy of *rajas*.

Remember as you set off to live your values and implement E2, these forces will still be at play. There will be times when it seems like just too much work to live E2 (*tamas*). There will be moments when you feel divinely inspired to do the inner work (*sattwa*). And there will be occasions when you just make yourself do what needs to be done (*rajas*). Know that the moods are a cycle, not an absolute.

Forget the people who say you can't do this or that, including your own self-deprecating voice. Remember that what you have chosen as an important value is indeed important. Focus your attention on role models—people that have successfully traveled where you'd like to be. Allow that to be your inspiration to continue on the inner work.

The Mind of a Cannibal

Speaking with a past coworker, I learned that 3,000 people were laid off from the company I used to work for. Whether organizational instability comes from a sinking economy, mergers or acquisitions, or re-engineering efforts, the results are the same: stress and anxiety for you as you try and do your job, balance work and family, and have a life in uncertain times.

Your response to instability can range from mild anxiety to full blown panic. Perhaps the most difficult time to practice making a conscious choice with your actions in E2 is when it feels like your body is in a fight or flight response, and the mind just keeps running nonstop with the stress of it all. An ancient story may give us a clue about how to live with more ease in difficult times.

Angulimala was a vicious cannibal living at the time of Buddha. Angulimala was on a mission to kill and then cut off the small fingers of 1,000 people, which he strung in a gruesome garland around his neck. When he had only one more finger to get to finish his nasty chore, Buddha arrived on the scene. Rather than run from Angulimala, Buddha said, "Come here, you are welcome." Angulimala ran and ran but could not catch Buddha, who was serenely walking. Exhausted and frustrated, Angulimala yelled to Buddha, "Stop!"

Buddha replied, "I have stopped. It is you who has to stop." With this, Angulimala's mind was transformed and he dropped his sword.

We all have worries that threaten to gobble us up whole. We either fight the anxiety, thinking that it should be other than it is, or we try to flee, thinking that we can safely exist only far away from the threat. But no matter how far we run, our mind is right there with us, keeping anxiety levels high. No matter how hard we fight, it only serves to create upheaval and inner tension as we try to "fix" what is wrong. Our mind can be our personal Angulimala, threatening to gobble us up with churning thoughts.

The next time you feel consumed by worry, tossing and turning at night, try a new approach. Accept the worry, welcoming it. Let's face it; the worry is there, so you might as well see it for what it is. Accept the worry, the uncertainty, the unknown.

Then, just as Buddha told Angulimala, stop. Stop trying to understand. Stop trying to control the situation. Stop trying to figure it all out. Stop wishing that others would behave differently. Stop weaving stories about the future. Stop trying to implement E2. Just stop. If only for a second, just stop trying to find a solution to your problem. Then the mind that has been chasing you, threatening to devour your peace, bows down.

Kim's Sunday

The other morning I attended a memorial service for a friend that died a year ago. She was in her late thirties and left behind a husband and two sons, ages three and ten.

Kim went to see her doctor on a Friday afternoon with symptoms of fatigue and bruising on her arm, attributing it to the recent birth of her son. That night the doctor called her at home and said she needed to see a specialist the next day. On Saturday Kim was told she had an aggressive form of leukemia and spent the day at the hospital having tests done. Although they usually admit people right away with this diagnosis, the doctor said he would give Kim a reprieve and wait until Monday to start treatment.

I wonder, what was Sunday like for Kim and her family?

As I was driving home late the same night of the memorial service, my mind was busy with all that I had to do. Like a record player, I was reviewing over and over again the projects I was involved in and what I needed to do.

All of a sudden I thought of Kim's Sunday. How important was her list of things to do when she realized she would be fighting for her life in the hospital the next day? What was the priority for her on that Sunday?

As I thought of this, I was able to let go of the tasks that made my gut tight and my mind worrisome. If none of it got done, it would not be the end of the world.

E2 is the ability to remember your values and choose them over and over and over again.

Keeping life's priorities top of mind may be a challenge when everyday responsibilities seem all consuming. Try looking at today as if it were Kim's Sunday. Are you living the life that's important to you? Do you know what's important to you?

Summary

- E2 stands for Elect or choose. It answers the question "How do I want to be in this moment?" It's taking the theory of your passion words and applying it to your day-to-day actions.

- Remember that you already possess all you need to live deliberately. Like making maple syrup, the process of E2 is just the continual action of boiling off what you don't need.

- Understanding the nature of your thoughts can help you transcend their power, enabling you to connect with a more permanent and positive aspect of being.

- When you are trying to live your values in E2, accept the fact that it will be messy. Trust the process and know that a new pattern will emerge for you.

- Your own self-defeating thoughts and the negative position of others can be a roadblock to your success in E2. Overcome this by finding a mentor or role model who you can emulate, and pay particularly strong attention to your own positive self-talk.

- If all else fails when trying to implement E2, just stop. Rest. In quiet and non-striving, peace can be found, enabling you to re-enter the world with new perspectives on E2.

- Keep your passion statement alive everyday by reminding yourself that life is finite.

- Life gives you plenty of opportunities to choose how you want to be in every moment. Take advantage of the opportunity by experimenting with E2.

The Footprint of Your Life

Life is not like taking a walk through a forest with an accurate compass, knowing exactly where you're going and how you'll get there. Life is more like walking through a long, high labyrinth. A labyrinth is a circular path that will, if you just keep walking, bring you to the center. While walking in a labyrinth you may feel disoriented, lost and alone, but you're not. Wherever you are leads you to the center. All you have to do is keep walking.

I walked in a labyrinth once. Not a tall grand one, but a small humble herb garden. As I walked, another person and I brushed shoulders. At the time we connected, I was looking down as my foot made contact with the earth. As my heel, then arch, then toes touched the path, I realized that this footprint was completely unique. Never before seen, never again to be experienced as it is, even by me. It was wholly, completely, its own, created by the relationship of my foot to the ground. Never before has anything interacted with the ground in this same manner, never again will it be repeated. Some might walk a similar, or even an identical path—I might even walk it again—but the experience was unique. It did not belong to me. It was a combination of interactions among pieces. The moment was a dance of parts creating a whole: the blade of grass, the dirt, my foot, the surrounding air, the sun that shone upon it. For me it was sacred, never to be again as it was then.

The realization held a responsibility: the footprint of each moment in my life was mine to value or not.

There's a wonderful Buddhist story about how precious your human life is. Imagine a huge ocean that covers the expanse of the earth. On the surface of the ocean floats an insignificant hoop, tiny in comparison to the vast water. In the ocean lives a turtle that surfaces once every 100 years to take a breath. The chance of you being born is the same chance as that turtle surfacing through the hoop to take his 100-year breath. If you lived as though your life were that precious and special, how would you go about your day?

The documentary of Buckminster Fuller, *Thinking Out Loud,* tells the story of this genius who invented the geodesic dome (the engineering feat of his time). In his mid twenties he went through an incredibly difficult period. His only daughter had died when she was still a toddler, and he was drinking heavily to deal with the pain. He was contemplating suicide near a lake one evening. As he looked out over the water, he realized he could not kill himself. He had collected certain knowledge that was wholly his own, his footprint in this world. As such, he could not kill himself, as it was his obligation to share it with others.

You have your own footprint that is being created right now. It's being created every moment of your life. Your footprint in the world is being created every time you take a breath, every time you make a choice, every time you smile, and every time you frown.

Exploring your own footprint of life is not separate from the act of creation. Simply by exploring your life, you create it. By consciously creating your life, you explore possibilities. Exploration and creation are not mutually exclusive; they are co-conspirators of your reality.

In this book I've presented a process to help you know your own footprint, to help you see the relationship between your explorations and your creations. The process looks neat, orderly, sequential and linear. It's not.

Take comfort in the fact that even though you might not know where you're going, or even how you got here, where you are contains your divine footprint.

In Yoga, Self with a capital "S" denotes the divinity within. The self with a small "s" is the ego self, the self of labels, positions, job, and roles. The Self is infinity. The self is the box. When it comes to seeing infinity in a box, the ancient poet and mystic Rumi says, "Work in the invisible world at least as hard as you do in the visible."

The invisible world is within you. Swami Muktananda, Siddha Yoga Master, said:

> *Meditate on your Self.*
> *Honor your Self.*
> *Worship your Self.*
> *Understand your own Self.*
> *God dwells within you as you.*

Let me finish this book the same way I finish my Yoga class. I put my hands together in a prayer position near my heart, bow to you, and say "Namaste," a word that means I bow to the light within you.

When you're in that light, and I'm in that light, we are one.

Resources

Bennett-Goleman, Tara. *Emotional Alchemy, How the Mind can Heal the Heart.* New York, NY: Three Rivers Press, 2001.

Childre, Doc and Howard Martin, with Donna Beech. *The Heartmath Solution.* HarperSanFrancisco, 1999.

Cope, Stephen. *Yoga and the Quest for the True Self.* New York, NY: Bantam Books, 1999.

Feuerstein, Georg. *The Shambhala Guide to Yoga.* Boston, MA: Shambhala, 1996.

Gyatso, Geshe Kelsang. *The Meditation Handbook.* London, England: Tharpa Publications, 1999.

————. *Introduction to Buddhism.* London, England: Tharpa Publications, 2001.

————. *Eight Steps to Happiness.* London, England: Tharpa Publications, 2001.

————. *Introduction to Buddhism.* London, England: Tharpa Publications, 2001.

Handy, Charles. *The Age of Unreason.* Boston, MA: Harvard Business School Press, 1990.

McAfee, John. *Into the Heart of Truth, The Spirit of Relational Yoga.* Woodland Park, CO: Woodland Publications, 2001.

Muktananda, Swami. *Where Are You Going?* South Fallsburg: NY, SYDA Foundation, 1994.

———. *Kundalini, The Secret of Life.* South Fallsburg, NY: SYDA Foundation, 1994.

Prabhavanda, Swami and Christopher Isherwood. *How to Know God, The Yoga Aphorisms of Patanjali.* The Vedanta Society of Southern California: Vedanta Press, 1981.

Stoler-Miller, Barbara. *Yoga, Discipline of Freedom.* New York, NY: Bantam Books, 1998.

Tart, Charles T. *Open Mind, Discriminating Mind: Reflections on Human Possibilities.* iUniverse.com, 2000.

Thoreau, Henry David. *Walden.* Philadelphia, PA: Courage Books, 1990.

Whyte, David. *The Heart Aroused, Poetry and the Preservation of the Soul in Corporate America.* New York, NY: Doubleday, 1994.

About the Author

Megan McDonough is a business yogini—helping people work and live with ease using introspective Yoga techniques. Drawing on her personal experience of more than 15 years in the corporate world and more than 10 years practicing Yoga, Megan helps people develop self-leadership—the ability to cultivate an inner strength irrespective of outer challenges and stresses.

The former president of the Central Massachusetts American Society for Training and Development, Megan is now president of her own company, Megan R. McDonough Company. She writes, teaches, coaches and consults about techniques for greater freedom and less tension. Additionally, Megan is editor and publisher of *A Minute for Me*, an e-newsletter for time-challenged people who choose to make living mindfully a priority. For a free subscription, go to www.urinfinityinabox.com.

Megan lives on a small farm in Massachusetts with her husband, their two children, and a black lab named Belle, happily making maple syrup.

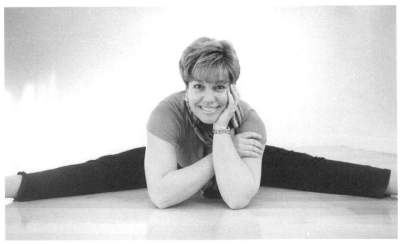

Photo by Susan Paquet